Empowering Youth: End HIV/AIDS

Nicholas

CONTENTS

PART A: RESEARCH PROTOCOL...1

Introduction ....2.

    Risk factors/determinants of HIV among AGYW...

    Interventions aimed at AGYW ....

    HIV testing services (HTS) ....

    Facilitators/determinants of HTS...

    Barriers of HTS...

Rationale...

Aims and Objectives ....

Methods for the 2012 South African National HIV Household survey..............................

    Study design ....

    Study population..

    Inclusion Criteria ....

    Exclusion Criteria ....

    Sampling, Recruitment & Enrolment for the main study..

    Research procedures and data collection methods ....

    Reliability and validity of tools ....

    Data Management and data analysis...

Methods for this sub-study of the 2012 South African National HIV Household survey ......

    Study design ....

    Study population..

    Exclusion Criteria ....

    Sampling...

    Data analysis...

    Ethical considerations ....

References ....

PART B: LITERATURE REVIEW 20

    Cultural risk factors..

    Socio-behavioural risk factors..

    Structural risk factors ....

    SES and Education..

References ....

PART C: MANUSCRIPT 30

Introduction 31

Objectives ....

Methods ....

    Study design and sample for the parent study ....

    Study design and sample for the sub-study ....

    Measures ....

    Statistical analysis ....

Results ....

    Summary of Demographic variables ....

    Associations with HIV Knowledge ....

    Logistic Regression Analysis ....

    Multivariate Regression Analysis ....

Discussion ....

Conclusion ....

Table legend ....

References ....

Tables ....

Appendices ....60.

PART A: RESEARCH PROTOCOL

Introduction

While much progress has been made in the fight against HIV/AIDS, the global epidemic remains a huge challenge. In 2016, there were approximately 36.7 million living with HIV and 1.8 million new infections worldwide (UNAIDS, 2017). A greater proportion (52%) of adults living with HIV, have been shown to be women in their reproductive age (15- 49 years). A third of new HIV infections occurred in young people aged 15-24 years although this population only makes up 10% of the total global population (UNAIDS, 2017). There are considerable differences in the number of new HIV infections between young men and women aged 15-24 years; with studies showing that 44% more of the new HIV infections occurring in women vs. in men in the same age group (UNAIDS, 2017). These figures illustrate that women are disproportionately more affected by HIV than men in this age group.

HIV is the second leading cause of death for adolescent girls and young women (AGYW) aged 15-24 years in Africa. Eastern and Southern Africa accounted for more than half (53%) of the global epidemic in 2016. Of this, Sub-Saharan Africa (SSA) account for approximately two thirds of new infections, of which 43% of new infections being across Eastern and Southern Africa (UNAIDS, 2017).

Dellar, Dlamini and Karim (2015) reported an incidence rate of 30% for AGYW in Southern Africa; signifying that AGYW contribute approximately 30% of all new infections in Southern Africa. It is therefore evident that Eastern and Southern Africa carries the heaviest burden.

While there have been significant advancements and progress made in the fight against HIV over the past decade to reduce the HIV transmission risk in South Africa, the country remains home to the highest number of people living with HIV (7.1 million) in the world (Shishana et al., 2014; UNAIDS, 2017). Of these, 270 000 are new infections, 100000 (37%) are made up by AGYW age 15-24 years (Johnson, Chiu, Myer, Davies, Dorrington, Bekker et al., 2016).

According to the 2012 South African National Household survey (SABSSM IV), the prevalence of HIV in youth aged 15-24 years was 7.1%. In a study by Dellar et al. (2015) and Harrison, Colvin, Kuo, Swartz and Lurie (2015) a disaggregation of their data showed that the prevalence of HIV among young women aged 20-24 years is higher in comparison to adolescent girls aged 15-19 years. Almost a quarter (24.1%) of all new HIV infections reported in the SABSSM IV survey occurred in AGYW aged 15-24 years (Shishana et al., 2014). AGYW had the highest incidence of HIV of 2.5%, which was over four times higher than the incidence rate found in males (0.6%) of the same age group (Shishana et al., 2014).

The disproportionality in the HIV incidence of young women compared to young men in the corresponding age group may be attributed to the age-sex disparity in the HIV infection rates. This implies that the age at which males and females get infected with HIV are as result of differing ages in the onset of sexual debut between them. Indicative of this is that young females are infected approximately 5-7 years earlier than young males, which often coincides with early sexual debut among females (Kharsany & Karim, 2016; Dellar, et al., 2015). Thus, the age-sex disparity in the transmission of HIV is sustained and plays a contributing role to the disproportionate burden of HIV in young females compared to young males (Dellar, et al. 2015). With this background, young females aged 15-24 years are thus considered a key population in HIV research. This implies that although attention ought to be placed on AGYW, more attention ought to be placed on young women aged 20-24 years when considering HIV and its associated risk factors.

Risk factors/determinants of HIV among AGYW

The disproportionate burden of HIV among young women may be attributed to a number of factors, which may increase vulnerability in this population group. Although the cause of HIV vulnerability in AGYW is not completely explained, there is an underlying interplay among biological, socio-behavioural and contextual factors, which has been associated with the rate of new HIV infections (Zuma et al., 2016; Dellar et al., 2015). Vulnerability to HIV may be due to a number of factors, which may include sexual or domestic violence, gender inequalities and biological differences as well. Differential access to health services may also be some of the reasons to explain the differences in the HIV burden between young men and women (Zuma et al., 2016). It has therefore been shown that women, particularly young women are more vulnerable to HIV, and this vulnerability corresponds to the higher rate of infections among young people. HIV is acquired by these AGYW mainly through heterosexual transmission (Dellar et al., 2015; Celum et al, 2015, Zuma et al., 2016). The interplay among biological, socio-behavioural and contextual factors is associated with the high rate of new HIV infections in this population group (Dellar, et al., 2015; Celum et al, 2015, Zuma et al., 2016). Additional risk factors for HIV transmission include; biological factors such as sexually transmitted infections; socio-behavioural factors such as having unprotected sex, multiple sex partners, being exposed to sexual violence as well as contextual factors such as high levels of migration and wealth disparities (Zuma et al, 2016).

Sociodemographic factors such as age, level of education, marital status and place of residence have been associated with HIV transmission risk among young people (Glynn et al., 2004; Doyle, Mavedzenge, Plummer & Ross, 2012). Poverty and residency have been reported as a contributing factor; as well as rural compared to urban residency such that HIV prevalence is higher in rural compared to urban areas (Steinert, Cluver, Melendez-Torres and Romero, 2016). This means that in poor households, there may be an expectation on AGYW to provide for themselves and their families, hence preventing them from staying in school (Mbirimtengerenji, 2007; Mufune 2014). As a result of the lack of or limited education, this has a strong influence on their decision to engage in unsafe sexual practices (Glynn et al., 2004; Doyle et al, 2012).

These risk factors, particularly for AGYW are as a result of societal norms which favours male dominance and sexual privilege which in turn leads to unequal power dynamics and gender inequality, creating an unfavourable environment for young females to negotiate safe sex (UNAIDS, 2016). This may subsequently lead them to engage in risky sexual behaviours (Niëns & Lowery, 2009; Wilson, Wright, Safrit & Rudy, 2010). Among AGYW, risky sexual behaviours associated with HIV infection include multiple sexual partnerships, early sexual debut, intimate partner violence, limited condom use, intergenerational and transactional sex (Pettifor et al., 2005; Pettifor, MacPhail, Rees & Cohen, 2008; Jewkes, Dunkle, Nduna & Shai, 2010; Stöckl, Kalra, Jacobi & Watts 2013; Kalichman, Simbayi, Kaufma, Cain, Jooste, 2007).

Interventions aimed at AGYW

South Africa has, over the past five years intensified interventions targeted at vulnerable groups such as AGYW (SANAC, 2018). Interventions or prevention strategies aimed at reducing the risk of HIV infection through sexual transmission among AGYW include the intensive promotion of female and male condoms, encouraging abstinence or delayed from sexual activity, the promotion of voluntary male medical circumcision, and antiretroviral therapy (ART) use (Thomson, Baeten, Mug, Bekker, Celum & Heffron, 2016). Most of these interventions rely heavily on the cooperation of the male partner or includes prevention for both young males and females (Thomson, Baeten, Mug, Bekker, Celum & Heffron, 2016).

Additional interventions such as pre-exposure prophylaxis (PrEP) are emerging interventions targeted particularly at high-risk populations (Thomson et al., 2016). PrEP is a recommended prevention strategy for people at high risk of HIV infection (WHO, 2012). Although these prevention strategies are forms of agency, control and empowerment, women at high risk of HIV infection lack delivery of PrEP. The lack of delivery of PrEP is due to clinical factors (i.e. low assessment of the efficacy of PrEP by clinical trial) and logistical factors (i.e. limited availability of antiretroviral medication, costs, infrastructure, and policies). These factors subsequently limit the scaling up of PrEP in high HIV burden areas and may be a result of the stigmatisation of HIV (Thomson et al, 2016; Dellar et al., 2015). In their study, Celum et al. (2015) found that daily PrEP uptake to be the highest form of protection for African AGYW. However, adherence thereof was reported to be low.

Additional interventions or prevention initiatives aimed at AGYW in South Africa are DREAMS (Determined Resilient Empowered AIDS-Free Mentored and Safe) and She Conquers campaign (PEPFAR, 2017). These initiatives are aimed at empowering AGYW through reducing new infections in AGYW in Sub-Saharan (SSA) countries, including South Africa. The main objectives are to reduce new infections in AGYW, reduce teenage pregnancies, increase retention in school until grade 12/matric, reduce sexual and gender-based violence, and to increase economic opportunities for young people. This is deemed achievable through evidence-based interventions (HIV testing, contraceptive, ante and postnatal services, post-violence care, parenting/caregiver, treatment and adherence programs, youth development, economic empowerment programmes). The intervention aims to address structural drivers (poverty, gender inequality, sexual violence, and lack of education) which increase the risk of AGYW contracting HIV. These initiatives target AGYW together with their male partners.

HIV testing services (HTS)

Even though HIV testing services, previously known as or referred to as HIV counselling and testing (HCT), have expanded dramatically, globally, approximately 3 in 10 of people living with HIV remain unaware of their HIV infection status (UNAIDS, 2017). Furthermore, the main approach aimed at reducing the spread of HIV infection in South Africa, is HIV testing services (HTS) (Pelter & Matseke, 2003). HTS is widely available at public health facilities in South Africa, and further available through non-medical sites as well as mobile services as to encompass a complete range of services to be provided with HIV testing.

In the 2012 South African National Household survey, among the young people aged 15-24 years, 52.2% among those that were sexually active reported having had an HIV test (60.1% females, 39.9% males). The HTS uptake was 63.6% (80.5% females' vs 47.7% males). The overall uptake of 52.2% is low given that there is increased availability of HTS services and an increase in HIV testing promotion campaigns countrywide. The relatively low uptake of HTS may mean that young people are not accessing the HTS services that could be effective in reducing their risk of HIV infection. Thus, it would be important to understand the reasons for this low uptake, particularly among females, in order to improve uptake in young people.

Facilitators/determinants of HTS

There are a number of factors associated with HIV testing. Such factors include knowledge about HIV, talking to a parent/guardian about HIV/AIDS or having impregnated someone (MacPhail et al., 2008; MacPhail et al., 2009; Peltzer & Matseke, 2013; Strauss et al., 2015). Hence, the need for support from the community (friends and family), offering the HTS service at no cost, and having mobile stations which assists in reducing cost implications are potential predictors of willingness to undergo testing (MacPhail et al., 2008; MacPhail et al., 2009). The associated factors with HIV testing appear to be true for only older females in this age group of 15-24 years. This alludes to younger females in the age group of 15-24 years, being less informed about sexual issues. Thus, the importance of knowledge on HIV and testing (as a factor influencing HIV testing behaviour) cannot be over-emphasised. This is evident as sexual reproductive health education, counselling, and provision of contraceptives is effective at increasing knowledge on sexual reproductive health (Salam et al., 2016). On the contrary, a lack of knowledge can be a major barrier to testing (Strauss, Rhodes & George, 2015).

Barriers of HTS

The perception of high risk of infection due to participating in risky sexual behaviour may also make young people less likely or more reluctant to test. On the contrary, persons not perceiving themselves as high risk due to perceived non-engaging in risky sexual activity were also less likely to undergo testing (Njagi & Maharaj, 2006). This corroborates the existing literature suggesting a relationship between risk perception and testing behaviour (Tenkorang, 2016).

Young people may therefore possibly refrain from undergoing HIV testing due to fear of discovering their HIV status regardless of risk perception. This fear may well be due to a lack of knowledge on ways in which to cope with a positive result. A second type of fear acting as a barrier to HIV testing is that of HIV-related discrimination and stigma regardless of the test result, as the main concern is in fact the confidentiality of the test result (MacPhail et al., 2008). This is linked to trust of the HTS healthcare worker and doubt in the effectiveness and availability of HIV medication, which may hinder the willingness of young people to test for HIV (MacPhail, et al., 2008; Strauss et al. 2015). This could be particularly the case at centres close to where they live/reside, as they would not prefer their status be known. Therefore, lack of testing may be associated with the perception of lack of support from friends, family and the community and healthcare system or be due to a lack of knowledge and awareness about HIV and testing.

According to the HTS guidelines, both pre and post-test counselling is available to aid knowledge. It is thus imperative to understand whether the uptake in HTS services is taking place and to identify gaps in this uptake, if any. Another barrier for young people, particularly for those of school going age is the delivery of health services, mainly access to these services. It is often difficult for young people to access these services. The difficulty is due to the opening hours of the facilities which overlaps with school going hours, the travel time as facilities are quite a distance from their place of residence, long queues prior to being attended to, cost implications as a result of transport or service fees and issues around consent for minors. Among minors (aged <18 years), ethical issues such as confidentiality and adult consent may also act as a barrier to accessing HIV testing services. All of these factors are limitations to accessing HTS services, which causes learners to miss school.

Although progress has been made towards fighting HIV through various interventions, it is imperative that prevention strategies be aligned with the associated risk factors for HIV in order to better understand the uptake or lack of these intervention strategies. There is therefore a need to understand and for a further scale up of targeted HIV interventions, particularly among AGYW in high HIV burden areas particularly.

Rationale

Although young females aged 15-24 years have been identified as a key population group at higher risk of HIV exposure and infection than other groups, information on their knowledge, and perceptions about HIV and how this impacts sexual and testing behaviour remains incomplete. There is a need to understand the determinants of HIV testing behaviour and sexual behaviour in order to inform appropriate targeted interventions to address the high burden of HIV and high incidence in young people.

Using the South African National HIV Household survey, 2012 (SABSSM IV) (published 2014) data set (published February 2018), this study proposes to investigate issues around knowledge, perceptions and how this impacts HIV testing and sexual behaviour in this target population.

Aims and Objectives

The study aims to investigate knowledge and perceptions about HIV risk behaviours in females aged 15-24 years and to explore any associations with the engagement of these young women in HIV testing and prevention services. The study will further explore how perceptions and behaviour impacts HIV testing and sexual behaviour in the target study population.

The objectives of this study are to:

1. Describe knowledge and perceptions on HIV (transmission and prevention) among young women aged 15-24 years enrolled in the SABSSM IV survey.
2. Investigate the association between HIV testing and:
   a) Knowledge about HIV (transmission and prevention)
   b) Sociodemographic characteristics (SES, locality, province, HIV status)
   c) Behavioural characteristics (risk associated – marital status, perceived risk, last HIV test, awareness of status, number of sexual partners)
3. Analyse HIV status and:
   a) Knowledge about HIV (transmission and prevention)
   b) Sociodemographic characteristics (SES, locality, province, HIV status)
   c) Behavioural characteristics (risk associated – marital status, perceived risk, last HIV test, awareness of status, number of sexual partners)

Variables under investigation

Independent	Dependent	Covariates
HIV testing	The engagement in HIV prevention practices (i.e. HTS services, regular testing, number of sexual partners)	Covariates: social demographic characteristics (age, race, locality, province, SES – income) Knowledge of HIV transmission and prevention
HIV status		Awareness of HIV status and HIV testing HIV risk factors (i.e. sexual behaviour)

Summary of variables and its associated measurement from the questionnaire (adult questionnaire – see Appendix 3) used for this sub-study

Variable	Scale
Demographic information	
Age	Numerical - continuous
Gender	Categorical - binary
Race	Categorical - nominal
Locality	Categorical – nominal
Province	Categorical – nominal
Income	Categorical – nominal
HIV awareness and testing	
Do you know of a place nearby where you can get an HIV test?	Categorical – binary
Have you ever had an HIV test?	Categorical – binary
How long ago did you have your most recent HIV test?	Categorical – nominal

Have you been told/informed of the result of your most recent test?	Categorical – binary
Where did you get your most recent HIV test?	Categorical – nominal
During your most recent HIV test, did you have counselling before the HIV test?	Categorical – binary
During your most recent HIV test, did you have counselling after the HIV test?	Categorical – binary
What was the main reason for going for your last HIV test?	Categorical – nominal
Have you ever been tested for HIV as part of the HIV Counselling and Testing (HTS) campaign launched by the president in 2010?	Categorical – nominal
Knowledge of HIV transmission and prevention	
Can a person reduce the risk of HIV by having fewer sexual partners?	Categorical – nominal
Can HIV be transmitted from a mother to her unborn baby?	Categorical – nominal
Can the risk of HIV transmission be reduced by having sex with only one uninfected partner who has no other partners?	Categorical – nominal
Can a person get HIV by sharing food with someone who is infected?	Categorical – nominal
Can a person reduce the risk of getting HIV by using a condom every time he/she has sex?	Categorical – nominal
Can medical male circumcision reduce the risk of HIV infection in males?	Categorical – nominal
HIV risk factors	
In total, with how many different people have you had sexual intercourse in your lifetime?	Numerical
Overall, how many sexual partners did you have during the past 12 months?	Numerical

Methods for the 2012 South African National HIV Household survey

Study design

The design used a multistage stratified cluster sampling approach, in which everyone in a sampled household was invited to participate.

Study population

The study population included persons of all ages living in South Africa based on the household an individual data collected from the SABSSM IV survey. The survey is carried out approximately every 3 years (2002, 2005, 2008 and 2012) and includes the general South African population.

Inclusion Criteria

- All persons (of all ages) living in South African households or hostels

Exclusion Criteria

- persons staying in any institution such as educational institutions,
- old-age homes,
- hospitals, and
- uniformed-service barracks

Sampling, Recruitment & Enrolment for the main study

The SABSSM IV survey used 1000 census enumeration areas (EAs) which was selected from a database of approximately 100 000 EAs that is regularly updated. The EAs are as officially defined by the South African national statistical agency, Statistics South Africa (StatsSA), and have been validated and enumerated for population censuses (Stats SA, 2013).

The selection of EAs was stratified by province and locality type. In addition, race type was also used as a stratification variable. The selection of EAs formed the primary sampling units (PSUs), visiting points (VPs) or households was used as secondary sampling units (SSUs), all consenting members of the household was the ultimate sampling unit (USU). A systematic random sample of 15 VPs was selected from each of the 1000 EAs, yielding a total sample size of 15,000 households or VPs. The pre-selected households were identified using aerial maps and also with the aid of GPS instruments whenever necessary. Up to three visits were made to each selected household in order to ensure maximum participation.

Research procedures and data collection methods

Data collectors were recruited to match the languages and races of selected EAs throughout the country and trained to conduct the survey. An enrolled or staff nurse was responsible for collecting blood samples from infants.

Prior to visiting households, the supervisors first made contact with the relevant gatekeepers. All participating household members' demographic characteristics were listed on both the visiting point and individual questionnaire. All participating children born to the participating mother were linked to the mother's questionnaire using a unique questionnaire number.

Recruitment and participation was encouraged at multiple levels, namely national, community, individual and social in the following ways; national – inform and alert the public of the HIV epidemic which South Africa is facing and inform them of the survey taking place in which it gets an official launch and involved the mass media, community – through media and specific targeting of communities, individual – appeal to individuals at household level to participate, social media –using social media (i.e. Facebook, Twitter etc.).

Reliability and validity of tools

The questionnaire used in SABSSM IV was not a validated tool; however, it was adapted and reviewed by team members prior to administration.

Data Management and data analysis

In the 2012 survey data was captured using the Census and Survey Processing System (CSPro) software programme (developed by the United States Census Bureau, Macro International, and Serpro, S.A).

Before the data analysis was conducted, data was checked and verified for consistency. The final weights of the data were computed to ensure that the estimates of HIV incidence, prevalence, and other outcomes of interest are representative of the general population of South Africa (Shishana et al., 2014).

Ethical considerations

The original proposal was reviewed and approved by the HSRC Research Ethics and by both the CDC Division of Global HIV and TB and the Centre for Global Health prior to its implementation REC number: 5/17/11/10 (see Appendix 1).

Informed consent procedures

All persons who agreed to participate were required to provide written or verbal (where respondent was illiterate) consent (see Appendix 2). Parents and guardians of children under 18 years were asked to give informed consent/permission for inclusion of children in the survey and verbal assent was obtained from all children to give a specimen for HIV testing.

Fieldwork staff was trained in informed consent procedures to ensure that voluntary informed consent is obtained for all participants. The study adhered to the South African Children's Act of 2007.

Procedures to ensure confidentiality

Interviews were held either inside or outside of the house with each individual respondent. Efforts were made to avoid interference from other members of the household. In addition, no names of individuals were recorded either on the tracking forms or on specimens. Instead, barcodes were used to link the questionnaires and blood specimens. To ensure further confidentiality, data was analysed nationally, provincially, and by EA type and not by smaller geographic units.

Methods for this sub-study of the 2012 South African National HIV Household survey
Study design

This will be a sub-study of a cross-sectional, population-based household survey, which employed a multistage stratified cluster sampling approach.

Study population

This study population will include household and individual data for females aged 15-24 years who were living in South Africa at the time of SABSSM IV survey.

Inclusion Criteria

- data of female participants (aged 15-24 years) living in South Africa who were recruited into the SABSSM IV survey

Exclusion Criteria

- data of males who were recruited in the SABSSM IV survey
- data of females below 15 years of age living in South Africa that were recruited in the SABSSM IV survey
- data of females above 25 years of age living in South Africa that were recruited in the SABSSM IV survey

Sampling

The sample includes household and individual data for females aged 15-24 years recruited into the SABSSM IV survey conducted in South Africa, stratified by province and locality type and that had provided consent to participate in the study and for future use, will be used and analysed.

Research procedures and data collection methods

The SABSSM IV data will be adjusted to fit the aforementioned inclusion criteria and sample. After which the data will be analysed to the purpose of establishing whether there are associations with HIV testing and sexual behaviour through knowledge and perceptions about HIV among this age group.

Data analysis

The data that is being used in this study has been curated, such that it has been checked and verified for consistency and is therefore representative of the general population of South Africa.

In this study, basic descriptive analyses and graphical displays will be performed for data at both national and provincial levels as well as in selected districts. The relationships between demographic, social and behavioural factors, and HIV infection and other outcomes of interest as outlined in the objectives will be assessed and analysed.

Ethical considerations

<u>Risks and benefits</u>

There are minimal risks of harm and discomfort as this study involves secondary data analysis only.

<u>Procedures to ensure confidentiality</u>

The dataset was anonymized and does not include the names or barcodes (which was used during to link participants in the collection of the raw data) of the participants. Access to the dataset is controlled and is for use only by students and co-supervisors. Further access to and use of the dataset, requires a formal process of application to be lodged to the HSRC.

References

1. Celum, C. L., Moretlwe, S. D., McConnell, M, van Rooyen, H., Bekker, L. G., Kurth, A. Bukusi, E., Desmond, C., Morton, J & Baeten, J. M. (2015). Rethinking HIV prevention to prepare for oral PrEP implementation for young African women. *Journal of the International AIDS Society 2015, 18*, 20227.

2. Dellar, R.C.; Dlamini, S & Karim, Q. A. (2015). Adolescent girls and young women: key populations for HIV epidemic control. *Journal of the International AIDS Society, 18*, 64-70.

3. Doyle, A. M., Mavedzenge, S. N., Plummer, M. L., Ross, D. A. (2012). The sexual behaviour ofadolescents in sub-Saharan Africa: patterns and trends from national surveys. *Tropical Medicine & International Health, 17*, 796–807.

4. DREAMS South Africa fact sheet (2016).

5. Fako T. T. (2006). Social and psychological factors associated with willingness to test for HIV infection among young people in Botswana. *AIDS Care, 18*, 201–207.

6. Glynn, J. R., Carael, M., Buve, A., Anagonou, S., Zekeng, L., Kahindo, M., et al. (2004). Does increased general schooling protect against HIV infection? A study in four African cities. *Tropical Medicine & International Health, 9*, 4–14.

7. Harrison, A., Colvin, C. J, Kuo, C., Swartz, A., & Lurie, M.. (2015). Sustained high HIV incidence in young women in southern Africa: social, behavioral and structural factors and emerging intervention approaches. *Current HIV/AIDS Reports, 12*, 207–15.

8. Jewkes, R. K., Dunkle, K., Nduna, M., & Shai, N. (2010). Intimate partner violence, relationship power inequity, and incidence of HIV infection in young women in South Africa: a cohort study. *Lancet, 376*, 41–48.

9. Johnson, L.F, Chiu, C., Myer, L., Davies, M., Dorrington, R.E., Bekker, L., et al. (2016). Prospects for HIV control in South Africa: a model-based analysis. *Global Health Action, 9*, 30314.

10. Kharsany, A. B. M. & Karim, Q. A. (2016). HIV Infection and AIDS in Sub-Saharan Africa: Current Status, Challenges and Opportunities. *The Open AIDS Journal, 10*, 34-48.

11. Kalichman, S. C., Simbayi, L. C., Kaufma, M., Cain, D., & Jooste, S. (2007). Alcohol use and sexual risks for HIV/AIDS in sub-Saharan Africa: systematic review of empirical findings. *Prevention Science, 8*, 141–151.

12. MacPhail, C. L., Pettifor, A., Coates T., Rees, H. (2008). 'You must do the test to know your status': attitudes to HIV voluntary counseling and testing for adolescents among South African youth and parents. *Health Education & Behavior, 35*, 87–104.

13. MacPhail, C., Pettifor, A., Moyo, W., Rees, H (2009). Factors associated with HIV testing among sexually active South African youth aged 15–24 years. *AIDS Care, 2*, 41 –67.

14. Mbirimtengerenji, N. D. (2007). Is HIV/AIDS Epidemic Outcome Of poverty in sub-Saharan Africa? *Croatian Medical Journal, 48*, 605–17.

15. Mufune, P. (2014). Poverty and HIV/AIDS in Africa: specifying the connections. *Social Theory & Health, 1*, 1–29.

16. Niëns, L. & Lowery, D. (2009). Gendered epidemiology: sexual equality and the prevalence of HIV/AIDS in sub-Saharan Africa. *Social Science Quarterly,90*, 1134–1144.

17. Njagi, F., & Maharaj, P. (2006). Access to voluntary counselling and testing services: perspectives of young people. *South Africa Review of Sociology, 37*, 113–27.

18. Peltzer K. & Matseke G. (2013). Determinants of HIV testing among young people aged 18 – 24 years in South Africa. *African Health Science, 13*, 1012-1020.

19. PEPFAR (2017). *Annual report to congress.*

20. Pettifor, A. E., Rees, H. V., Kleinschmidt, I., Steffenson, A. E., MacPhail, C., Hlongwa-Madikizela, L, et al. (2005). Young people's sexual health in South Africa: HIV prevalence and sexual behaviors from a nationally representative household survey. *AIDS, 19*, 1525–1534.

21. Pettifor A, MacPhail C, Rees H & Cohen M. HIV and sexual behavior among young people (2008): the South African paradox. *Sexually Transmitted Diseases, 35*, 843–844.

22. SANAC (2018). Adolescent Girls and Young Women (AGYW) Summit. http://sanac.org.za/2018/04/20/adolescent-girls-and-young-women-agyw-summit-24-25-april-2018/

23. Salam, R.A., Faqqah, A, Sajjad, N., Lassi, Z. S. Das, J.K., Kaufman, M. Bhutta, Z.A. (2016). Improving Adolescent Sexual and Reproductive Health: A Systematic Review of Potential Interventions. *Journal of Adolescent Health, 59*, 11- 28.

24. Shisana, O., Rehle, T., Simbayi, L. C., Zuma, K., Jooste, S., Zungu, N., Labadarios, D., Onoya, D. et al. (2014) *South African National HIV Prevalence, Incidence and Behaviour Survey, 2012*. Cape Town, HSRC Press.

25. Stats SA (Statistics South Africa) (2013) Mid-year population estimates.

26. Strauss, M. Rhodes, B. & George, G. (2015). A qualitative analysis of the barriers and facilitators of HIV counselling and testing perceived by adolescents in South Africa. *BMC Health Services Research, 5,* 1-12.

27. Stöckl, H., Kalra, N., Jacobi, J., & Watts, C.(2013). Is early sexual debut a risk factor for HIV infection among women in sub-Saharan Africa? A systematic review. *American Journal of Reproductive Immunology, 69,* 27–40.

28. Steinert, J. I., Cluver, L., Melendez-Torres, G. J. & Romero, R. H. (2016): Relationships between poverty and AIDS Illness in South Africa: an investigation of urban and rural households in KwaZulu-Natal, Global Public Health, DOI: 10.1080/17441692.2016.1187191

29. Szwarcwalda, C. L., Barbosa-Ju´niorb, A., Pascomb, A. R. & de Souza-Ju´niora, P.R. (2005). Knowledge, practices and behaviours related to HIV transmission among the Brazilian population in the 15–54 years age group. *AIDS, 19,* 51–58.

30. Tenkorang, E. Y. (2016). Perceived vulnerability and HIV testing among youth in Cape Town, South Africa. *Health Promotion International, 31,* 270–279.

31. Thomson, K. A., Baeten, J. M., Mugo, N. R., Bekker, L.G. Celum, C. L. & Heffron, R. (2016). Tenofovir-based Oral PrEP Prevents HIV Infection among Women. *Current Opinion in HIV and AIDS, 11,* 18-26.

32. UNAIDS. (2015).

33. Global AIDS update 2016: fast-tracking the response in eastern and southern Africa – focus on Adolescent Girls & Young Women. Global AIDS update 2016, and prevention gap report, UNAIDS, Geneva; 2016. Geneva: UNAIDS.

34. UNAIDS. *UNAIDS 2016-2021 Strategy*; August 2015.

35. UNAIDS (2016). HIV prevention among adolescent girls and young women: putting HIV intervention among adolescent girls and young women on the fast-track and engaging men and boys. Geneva: UNAIDS.

36. UNAIDS. *Global AIDS Update 2017;* July 2017. UNAIDS. *AIDSinfo website*; accessed July 2017, available at: http://aidsinfo.unaids.org/. UNAIDS. *Core Epidemiology Slides*; June 2017.

37. UNAIDS. *Fact Sheet 2017*; July 2017.

38. UNAIDS. *Core Epidemiology Slides*; June 2017.

39. Wilson, C.M., Wright. P. F., Safrit, J.T. & Rudy, B. (2010). Epidemiology of HIV infection and risk in adolescents and youth. *Journal of Acquired Immune Deficiency Syndrome, 54,* S5-S6.

40. World Health Organization. Guidance on pre-exposure oral prophylaxis (PrEP) for serodiscordant couples, men and transgender women who have sex with men at high risk of HIV: Recommendations for use in the context of demonstration projects. Geneva: 2012. http://www.who.int/hiv/pub/guidance_prep/en/).

41. Yaya, S. Bishwajit, G, Danhoundo, G, Shah, V. & Ekholuenetale, M. (2016). Trends and determinants of HIV/AIDS knowledge among women in Bangladesh. *BMC Public Health, 6,* 1-9.

42. Zuma, K., Shisana, O., Rehle, T. M., Simbayi, L.C., Jooste, S., Zungu, N., Labadarios, D., Onoya, D., Evans, M., Moyo, S. & Abdullah, F. (2016). New insights into HIV epidemic in South Africa: key findings from the National HIV Prevalence, Incidence and Behaviour Survey. *African Journal of AIDS Research, 15,* 67-75.

PART B: LITERATURE REVIEW

While much progress has been made, HIV remains a major global public health problem. In 2018, an estimated 37.9 million people worldwide were living with HIV, of which 20.6 million were living in Eastern and Southern Africa (UNAIDS, 2019). Globally, South Africa has the highest number of people living with HIV (7.9 million) an increase of 1.6 million since the 2012 estimate (Simbayi et al., 2019).

HIV is a major concern among adolescent girls and young women (AGYW), particularly in South Africa as AGYW carry the highest burden of HIV infections. In 2017, AGYW accounted for 100 000 new infections and were 3 times at higher risk of HIV infection than their male counterparts (Simbayi et al., 2019). There are multidimensional factors that predispose AGYW to the risk of HIV infection. These include the interplay among cultural, structural and socio-behavioural factors (Dellar, Dlamini & Karim, 2015; Celum et al, 2015; Zuma et al., 2016).

Cultural risk factors

A widespread patriarchal societal norm empowers and favours male dominance in South Africa (UNICEF, 2012). This power imbalance creates disparities and enables men to feel sexually entitled through the refusal of having to partake in safe sex practices, while placing AGYW in unfavourable conditions making them unable to negotiate safe sex (UNAIDS, 2016). These cultural norms have implications for both socio-behavioural and structural HIV risk factors among AGYW.

Socio-behavioural risk factors

AGYW are increasingly exposed to and having sex with men with a much higher HIV prevalence. Men in this age group (aged 20-30 years) (Bekker et al., 2015; UNICEF, 2017) compared to a younger group, are predisposed to HIV risk due the traditional patriarchal societal norms and gender attitudes which are closely linked to sexual practices. These sexual practices may increase exposure to intimate partner violence (IPV) and gender-based violence (GBV) linked to sexual violence, or may led to the engagement of risky sexual behaviours (i.e. the lack of or inconsistent condom use, sex while under the influence of alcohol, early sexual debut, multiple sexual partnerships, transactional sex, age-disparate sexual relationships) (Niëns & Lowery, 2009; Wilson, Wright, Safrit & Rudy, 2010; Stoner et al., 2019; Evans et al., 2016, 2017; Shishana et al., 2014; Pettifor et al., 2005; Pettifor, MacPhail, Rees & Cohen, 2008; Jewkes, Dunkle, Nduna & Shai, 2010; Stöckl, Kalra, Jacobi & Watts 2013; Kalichman,

Simbayi, Kaufma, Cain, Jooste, 2007, Simbayi et al., 2019). Socio-behavioural factors thus play a critical role in HIV infection among AGYW (Pettifor, Stoner, Pike, & Bekker, 2018; Simbayi et al., 2019).

Structural risk factors

The most crucial implication that traditional patriarchal societal norms have on AGYW is that of socio-economic status (SES), as women are often dependent on men for financial support and sustenance (Govender, Masebo, Nyamaruze, Cowden, Schunter & Bains, 2018). Low relative socio-economic status has been found to be associated with higher risk of HIV infection (Mbirimtengerenji, 2007; Mufune, 2014; Rodrigoa & Rajapakseb, 2010; Kalichman et al., 2004). These findings are well demonstrated by the association between SES and risky sexual behaviour, which illustrate that as a result of the significant economic pressures they face, women from poorer households were more likely to engage in risky sexual behaviour (i.e. transactional sex as one such example) than women from more affluent households (Booysen, 2004). Low relative socio-economic status may be attributed to high levels of poverty and inequality in South Africa and may result in unequal access to healthcare and education (Lopman, Lewis, Nyamukapa, Mushati, Chandiwana, Gregson; 2007; Sishana et al., 2014; UNAIDS, 2019b). Women with low SES were found to have greater limitations with accessing healthcare services than women from more affluent households (Shishana et al., 2014).

SES and Education

AGYW of low relative SES are expected to provide for themselves and their families. This not only places immense pressure on AGYW but also prevents them from remaining in school (Mbirimtengerenji, 2007; Mufune, 2014), making education a key factor to consider. Individuals with limited access to education have limited access to safe-sex information and this has a strong influence on their decision to engage in unsafe sexual practices (Gregson et al., 2004; Glynn et al., 2004; Doyle et al, 2012). By not adopting a protective lifestyle and behaviour, AGYW's vulnerability to HIV is increased (Gregson et al., 2004). Women from low relative SES were found to be less likely to be knowledgeable about HIV than women from affluent households (Booysen & Summerton, 2002).

Levels of HIV knowledge are also associated with more general levels of education. Research shows that as level of education increased, so did knowledge of HIV transmission (Chambers, Haile, Richardson & Richardson, 2002; Burgoyne & Drummond, 2008). Higher levels of education better prepares individuals to respond to HIV, as the knowledge of HIV that is provided is understood better at a higher level of education (Burgoyne & Drummond, 2008). Thus, the higher the education level the more protective effects it has against HIV for AGYW.

HIV knowledge among AGYW is generally low (UNAIDS, 2019a). Globally, only 23% of AGYW have correct knowledge of HIV (UNAIDS, 2019a). Only 31% of AGYW in sub-Saharan Africa have correct knowledge of HIV (UNAIDS, 2019a). This is of concern, as low knowledge is associated with higher HIV risk (Israel, Lauder & Simonetti, 2008). AGYW decision-making regarding engaging in unsafe sexual practices are strongly influenced by having low HIV knowledge (Glynn et al., 2004; Doyle et al, 2012). This is illustrated through having unsafe (condom-less) sex which may at times be due to a lack of HIV knowledge (Mavhu et al., 2018). This in turn predisposes AGYW to HIV risk.

Hence, having HIV knowledge may result in partaking in safer behaviours as to reduce their HIV risk. Knowledge of HIV thus equips individuals better to adopt to safe sexual practices and their respective sexual behaviour (Bertrand et al., 2006). Having HIV knowledge may also result in being aware of one's HIV status and perceived risk of HIV (Sherr et al., 2007; Tenkorang et al., 2009; Tenkorang & Maticka-Tyndale, 2013). Knowledge of HIV comes from various sources, such as sexual and reproductive health education and the experience of HIV counselling and testing (Sherr et al., 2007; Tenkorang et al., 2009; Tenkorang and Maticka-Tyndale, 2013).

HIV counselling and testing (HCT) is essential as it informs individuals of their HIV status, assists with HIV prevention strategies, enables HIV-positive individuals to receive the necessary care and treatment, and encourages HIV-negative individuals to maintain their status (Marks, Crepaz & Janssen, 2006; Tenkorang & Maticka-Tyndale, 2013; Peltzer, Matseke, Mzolo, & Majaja, 2009).

Lack of knowledge is an important barrier to testing. One barrier to testing is through fearfulness and denial. Lack of knowledge increases fearfulness and denial (Strauss, Rhodes and George, 2015). This in turn makes people susceptible to stigma and fear, both of which lowers HIV testing rates (Treves-Kagan et al., 2017; Parker & Aggleton, 2003). This is illustrated through the association found between the fear and stigma around an HIV positive result and delay in testing or the decision to get tested (Kalichman & Simbayi, 2003; Chesney

& Smith, 1999). Another barrier to testing is through lack of knowledge about how testing works and where it is available (i.e. testing sites) (Choi, Lui, Guo, Han, & Mandel, 2006). Therefore, not knowing about available services reduces HIV testing (Mohlabane, 2016).

Although solid HIV knowledge is critical for effective HIV prevention, there is a lack of knowledge among AGYW. This lack of knowledge is a risk for AGYW as it predisposes them to HIV infection. Better understanding the levels of HIV knowledge and how knowledge levels correlate with specific HIV risk factors is an important area of research. If we know more about this, we can improve the existing HIV prevention aimed at increasing the knowledge of AGYW and expand on the limited research in this area.

References

1. Bekker, L. G., Johnson, L. Wallace, M., Hosek, S. (2015). Building our youth for the future. *J Int AIDS Soc, 18*, 200-227.

2. Bertrand, J. B., O'Reilly, K., Denison, J. Anhang, R, Sweat, M. (2006). Systematic review of the effectiveness of mass communication programs to change HIV/AIDS-related behaviors in developing countries, *Health Education Research, 21*, 567–597.

3. Booysen Fle. R. (2004). HIV/AIDS, poverty and risky sexual behaviour in South Africa. *Afr J AIDS Res 3*, 57-67.

4. Booysen Fle., R. & Summerton, J. (2002). Poverty, risky sexual behaviour, and vulnerability to HIV infection: Evidence from South Africa. *J Health Popul Nutr., 20*, 285–288.

5. Burgoyne, A. D. & Drummond, P. D. (2008). Knowledge of HIV and AIDS in women in sub-Saharan Africa. *African Journal of Reproductive Health, 12,*14-31.

6. Celum, C. L., Moretlwe, S. D., McConnell, M, van Rooyen, H., Bekker, L. G., Kurth, A. Bukusi, E., Desmond, C., Morton, J & Baeten, J. M. (2015). Rethinking HIV prevention to prepare for oral PrEP implementation for young African women. *Journal of the International AIDS Society 2015, 18*, 20227.

7. Chambers, J., Haile, B., Richardson, A. richardson, C. (2001). Annual conference HIV?AIDS survey: analyses and implications. Annual Conference of the 19th Episcopal District of the African Methodist Episcopal District of the African Episcopal Church. Johannesburg, South Africa 2002.

8. Dellar, R. C, Dlamini, S. & Karim, Q. A. (2015). Adolescent girls and young women: key populations for HIV epidemic control. *Journal of the International AIDS Society, 18*, 64-70.

9. Doyle, A. M., Mavedzenge, S. N., Plummer, M. L., Ross, D. A. (2012). The sexual behaviour of adolescents in sub-Saharan Africa: patterns and trends from national surveys. *Tropical Medicine & International Health, 17*, 796–807.

10. Chesney, M.A. & Smith, A.W. (1999). Critical delays in HIV testing and care: the potential role of stigma. *Am Behav Sci.,42,* 1162–74.

11. Choi, K. H., Lui, H., Guo, Y., Han, L., & Mandel, J. S. (2006). Lack of HIV testing and awareness of HIV infection among men who have sex with men, Beijing, China. *AIDS Education and Prevention, 18*, 33-43.

12. Glynn, J. R., Carael, M., Buve, A., Anagonou, S., Zekeng, L., Kahindo, M., et al. (2004). Does increased general schooling protect against HIV infection? A study in four African cities. *Tropical Medicine & International Health, 9*, 4–14.

13. Govender, K., Masebo, W., Nyamaruze, P., Cowden, R. G., Schunter, B. T., & Bains, A. (2018). HIV Prevention in Adolescents and Young People in the Eastern and Southern African Region: A Review of Key Challenges Impeding Actions for an Effective Response. *The open AIDS journal, 12*, 53–67.

14. Gregson, S. Terceira, N., Mushati, P., Nyamukapa, C. Campbell, C. (2004). Community group participation: Can it help young women to avoid HIV? An exploratory study of social capital and school education in rural Zimbabwe. *Soc Sci Med, 58*, 2119–2132.

15. Israel, E., Laudar, C. & Simonetti, C. (2008). HIV prevention among vulnerable populations: Pathfinder International Technical Guidance Series Number 6.

16. Joint United Nations Programme on HIV/AIDS (UNAIDS). AIDSinfo. Geneva, Switzerland: UNAIDS; 2017. http://aidsinfo.unaids.org/

17. Kalichman S., Simbayi L. C. (2003) HIV testing attitudes, AIDS stigma, and voluntary HIV counseling and testing in a black township in Cape Town, South Africa. *Sexually Transmitted Infections, 79*, 442–447.

18. Kalichman, S. C., Simbayi, L. C., Kaufma, M., Cain, D., & Jooste, S. (2007). Alcohol use and sexual risks for HIV/AIDS in sub-Saharan Africa: systematic review of empirical findings. *Prevention Science, 8*, 141–151.

19. Karim. S.S.A., Churchyard. G.J., Karim, Q.A. & Lawn, S.D. (2010). HIV infection and tuberculosis in South Africa: an urgent need to escalate the public health response. *Lancet, 374*, 921–33.

20. Lopman, B., Lewis, J., Nyamukapa, C., Mushati, P., Chandiwana, S., Gregson S. (2007). HIV incidence and poverty in Manicaland, Zimbabwe: Is HIV becoming a disease of the poor? *AIDS, 21*, 57-66.

21. MacPhail, C., Pettifor, A., Moyo, W., & Rees, H. (2009). Factors associated with HIV testing among sexually active South African youth aged 15-24 years. *AIDS Care, 21*(4), 456-467.

22. Marks, G., Crepaz, N. & Janssen, R.S. (2006). Estimating sexual transmission of HIV from persons aware and unaware that they are infected with the virus in the USA. *AIDS, 20*,1447–50.

23. Maughan-Brown, B., & Venkataramani, A. S. (2017). Accuracy and determinants of perceived HIV risk among young women in South Africa. *BMC Public Health, 18*, 42.

24. Mavhu, W., Rowley, E., Thior, I., Kruse-Levy, N., Mugurungi, O., Ncube, G., et al. (2018). Sexual behavior experiences and characteristics of male-female partnerships among HIV positive adolescent girls and young women: Qualitative findings from Zimbabwe. *PLoS ONE 13*.

25. Meiberg, A. E., Bos, A. E. R., Onya, H. E., & Schaalma H. P. (2008) Fear of stigmatization as barrier to voluntary HIV counselling and testing in South Africa. *East African Journal of Public Health, 5*, 49–54.

26. Mbirimtengerenji, N. D. (2007). Is HIV/AIDS Epidemic Outcome Of poverty in sub-Saharan Africa? *Croatian Medical Journal, 48*, 605–17.

27. Mohlabane, N., Tutshana, B., Peltzer, K., Mwisongo, A. (2016). Barriers and facilitators associated with HIV testing uptake in South African health facilities offering HIV Counselling and Testing. *Health SA Gesondheid 21*, 86–95.

28. Mufune, P. (2014). Poverty and HIV/AIDS in Africa: specifying the connections. *Social Theory & Health, 1*, 1–29.

29. Niëns, L. & Lowery, D. (2009). Gendered epidemiology: sexual equality and the prevalence of HIV/AIDS in sub-Saharan Africa. *Social Science Quarterly,90,* 1134–1144.

30. Parker, R. & Aggleton, P. (2003). HIV and AIDS-related stigma and discrimination: a conceptual framework and implications for action. *Soc Sci Med.,57*, 13–24.

31. Peltzer, K., Matseke, G., Mzolo, T., & Majaja, M. (2009). Determinants of knowledge of HIV status in South Africa: results from a population-based HIV survey. *BioMedCentral Public Health, 9*, 174.

32. Peltzer, K. & Matseke G. (2013). Determinants of HIV testing among young people aged 18 – 24 years in South Africa. *African Health Science, 13,* 1012-1020.

33. Pettifor, A., MacPhail, C., Rees, H. & Cohen, M. (2008). HIV and sexual behavior among young people: The South African paradox. *Sexually Transmitted Diseases, 35*, 843–844.

34. Pettifor, A., Stoner, M., Pike, C., & Bekker, L. G. (2018). Adolescent lives matter: preventing HIV in adolescents. *Current opinion in HIV and AIDS, 13*, 265–273.

35. Salam, R.A., Faqqah, A., Sajjad, N., Lassi, S., Das, J.K., Kaufman, M. & Bhutta, Z. A. (2016). Improving Adolescent Sexual and Reproductive Health: A Systematic Review of Potential Interventions. *Journal of Adolescent Health, 59,*11-28.

36. Sherr, L., Lopman, B., Kakowa, M., Dube, S., Chawira G., Nyamukapa, C., et al. (2007). Voluntary counseling and testing: uptake, impact on sexual behavior, and HIV in a rural Zimbabwean cohort. *AIDS, 21*, 851–860.

37. Shisana, O., Rehle, T., Simbayi, L. C., Zuma, K., Jooste, S., Zungu, N., Labadarios, D., Onoya, D. et al. (2014). *South African National HIV Prevalence, Incidence and Behaviour Survey, 2012*. Cape Town, HSRC Press.

38. Simbayi, L.C., Zuma, K., Zungu, N., Moyo, S., Marinda, E., Jooste, S., Mabaso, M., Ramlagan, S., North, A., van Zyl, J., Mohlabane, N., Dietrich, C., Naidoo, I. and the SABSSMV Team. (2019). South African National HIV Prevalence, Incidence, Behaviour and Communication Survey, 2017. Cape Town: HSRC Press

39. South Africa National Department of Health (2015). National consolidated guidelines for the prevention of mother-to-child transmission of HIV (PMTCT) and the management of HIV in children, adolescents and adults. Pretoria: National Department of Health.

40. Spyrelis, A., Abdulla, S., Frade, S., Meyer, T., Mhazo, M., Taruberekera, N., Taljaard, D. & Billy, S. (2017). Are women more likely to self-test? A short report from an acceptability study of the HIV self-testing kit in South Africa. *AIDS Care, 29*,339-343.

41. Strauss, M. Rhodes, B. & George, G. (2015). A qualitative analysis of the barriers and facilitators of HIV counselling and testing perceived by adolescents in South Africa. *BMC Health Services Research, 5*, 1-12.

42. Stöckl, H., Kalra, N., Jacobi, J., & Watts, C. (2013). Is early sexual debut a risk factor for HIV infection among women in sub-Saharan Africa? A systematic review. *American Journal of Reproductive Immunology, 69*, 27–40.

43. Stoner, M.C.D., Nguyen, N., Kilburn, K. et al. (2019). Age-disparate partnerships and incident HIV infection in adolescent girls and young women in rural South Africa. *AIDS. 33*, 83-91.

44. Tenkorang, E. Y. & Maticka-Tyndale, E. (2013) Individual-and school- level correlates of HIV testing among secondary school students in Kenya. *Studies in Family Planning, 44*, 169–187.

45. Tenkorang, E.Y. (2016). Perceived vulnerability and HIV testing among youth in Cape Town, South Africa. *Health Promotion International, 31*,270–279.

46. Treves-Kagan, S., El Ayadi, A. M., Pettifor, A., MacPhail, C., Twine, R., Maman, S., Peacock, D., Kahn, K., & Lippman, S. A. (2017). Gender, HIV Testing and Stigma: The Association of HIV Testing Behaviors and Community-Level and Individual-

Level Stigma in Rural South Africa Differ for Men and Women. *AIDS Behav, 21,* 2579–2588.

47. UNAIDS, 2019a. Power to the people.

48. UNAIDS, 2019b. A spotlight on adolescent girls and young women.

49. UNICEF (2012). Thematic discussion on the work of UNICEF in humanitarian situations.

50. UNAIDS (2016). HIV prevention among adolescent girls and young women: putting HIV intervention among adolescent girls and young women on the fast-track and engaging men and boys. Geneva: UNAIDS.

51. UNICEF (2017). Children and AIDS: statistical update.

52. Upadhya, D., Moll, A. P., Brooks, R. P., Friedland, G., & Shenoi, S. V. (2016). What motivates use of community-based human immunodeficiency virus testing in rural South Africa? *International Journal Of STD & AIDS, 27*(8), 662-671.

53. Wilkinson, R. G. 1996. *Unhealthy Societies: The Afflictions of Inequality.* London: Routledge.

54. Wilkinson, R. G. 2000. *Mind the Gap: Hierarchies, Health, and Human Evolution.*

55. Wilson, C.M., Wright. P. F., Safrit, J.T. & Rudy, B. (2010). Epidemiology of HIV infection and risk in adolescents and youth. *Journal of Acquired Immune Deficiency Syndrome, 54,* S5-S6.

56. World Health Organization (2013). Global update on HIV treatment: results, impact and opportunities. Geneva: WHO Press.

57. Zuma, T., Seeley, J., Sibiya, L. O., Chimbindi, N., Birdthistle, I., Sherr, L., & Shahmanesh, M. (2019). The Changing Landscape of Diverse HIV Treatment and Prevention Interventions: Experiences and Perceptions of Adolescents and Young Adults in Rural KwaZulu-Natal, South Africa. *Frontiers in public health, 7,* 336.

PART C: MANUSCRIPT

Knowledge and perceptions about HIV among adolescent girls and young women aged 15-24 years: associations with HIV testing and sexual behaviour – a sub-study of the 2012 South African National HIV Household survey

F Frieslaar, BSocSc Hons [1]; C Colvin [2]; R Tadokera, PhD, MPH [3]; S Jooste [4]

[1] MPH Student School of Public Health and Family Medicine, University of Cape Town, South Africa.
[2] School of Public Health and Family Medicine, University of Cape Town, South Africa.
[3] NRF/DST Centre of Excellence for Biomedical Tuberculosis Research; South African Medical Research Council Centre for Tuberculosis Research; Division of Molecular Biology and Human Genetics, Faculty of Medicine and Health Sciences, Stellenbosch University, Cape Town, South Africa.
[4] Human Sciences Research Council.

Background. While much progress has been made, HIV remains a major global public health problem. South Africa remains home to the highest number of people living with HIV (7.1 million) in the world. Despite remarkable progress in the past decade, adolescent girls and young women aged 15-24 (AGYW) remain at higher risk of HIV exposure and infection than other groups. We do not know enough about AGYW HIV knowledge and perceptions, although it is likely an important factor to consider in AGYW's HIV risk. This paper investigates knowledge and perceptions about HIV risk behaviours and explores associations with demographic and behavioral characteristics among AGYW in South Africa.

Methods. This sub-study is based on the 2012 South African National HIV Prevalence, Incidence and Behaviour Survey, a cross-sectional population-based household survey. A multistage stratified cluster sampling approach was employed to select the study population. Multivariate logistic regression was used to determine associations or factors which were associated with HIV knowledge.

Results. Among the sample of 3700 AGYW aged 15-24 years, White [OR=2.44 (95% CI: 1.48-4.03), p=0.001] and Indian [OR=3.85 (95% CI: 2.39-6.18), p=0.000] AGYW were associated with high HIV knowledge compared to Black Africans. AGYW in urban informal [OR=0.64 (95% CI: 0.45-0.90), p=0.011] and rural informal [OR=0.57 (95% CI: 0.33-0.98), p=0.043] were associated with low HIV knowledge compared to urban formal settings.

AGYW in Eastern Cape [OR=0.69 (95% CI: 0.48-1.00), p=0.048], KwaZulu-Natal [OR=0.69 (95% CI: 0.48-0.99), p=0.044], North West [OR=0.50 (95% CI: 0.32-0.77), p=0.002] and Limpopo [OR=0.44 (95% CI: 0.27-0.71), p=0.001] provinces were associated with low HIV knowledge compared to AGYW in Western Cape. Unemployed AGYW were associated with low HIV knowledge [OR=0.57, p=0.001]. While AGYW with higher levels of education: grade 12 [OR=1.66 (95% CI: 1.04-2.64), p=0.034] and tertiary [OR=2.68 (95% CI: 1.47-4.89), p=0.001] were associated with high HIV knowledge. AGYW having had sex in the last 12 months were associated with high HIV knowledge [OR=1.70 (95% CI: 1.08-2.72), p=0.023]. On the contrary, having multiple sexual partners in the last 12 months was associated with low HIV knowledge [OR= 0.60 (95%CI: 0.39-0.99), p=0.045] compared to AGYW that had 1 sexual partner in the last 12 months. AGYW with a low risk of alcohol use were associated with high HIV knowledge [OR=1.4 (95% CI: 1.02-1.87), p=0.039] compared to AGYW that abstained from alcohol. The final multivariate logistic regression model showed that AGYW in urban informal settings have low HIV knowledge [aOR=0.59 (95% CI: 0.35-0.99), p=0.046] among all geotypes.

Conclusion. Overall, the main findings show a lack of knowledge among AGYW across race, geotype, province and sexual activity. More specifically that low HIV knowledge was associated with AGYW who were Black South Africans, living in informal settings, from Eastern Cape, KwaZulu Natal, North West and Limpopo, unemployed, had lower levels of education, and have multiple sexual partners. However, in the final multivariate analysis, only geotype stood out, indicating that there is an HIV knowledge deficit in urban informal settings. This can be addressed through the promotion of knowledge through education, equitable and accessible availability of education and sexual and reproductive health services, and HCT and support among AGYW living in urban informal settings.

Introduction

Globally, every week 6000 AGYW become infected with HIV, most being from Africa (UNAIDS, 2019). In Eastern and Southern Africa, the HIV prevalence among AGYW is more than double that of their male counterparts (UNAIDS, 2019). In South Africa, AGYW have the highest burden of new infections of HIV, accounting for approximately 100 000 new infections yearly (Simbayi et al., 2019). AGYW have the highest incidence among the total 88400 new infections, they make up 66 200 (1.51%) and young men make up 22 200 (0.49%) (Simbayi et al., 2019). AGYW in South Africa therefore have 3 times higher risk of HIV infection than their male counterparts and account for almost quarter of all new infections (Simbayi et al., 2019).

Several factors increase the risk of HIV infection among AGYW. These risk factors include age-disparate sexual relationships (an age gap of 5 years or more between partners), multiple sexual partners (MSP), exposure to sexual violence, alcohol use and risky sexual behaviour (i.e. inconsistent condom use or condom-less sex, transactional sex) (Shishana et al., 2014; Maughan-Brown et al., 2018; Simbayi et al., 2019; Stoner et al., 2019). The aforementioned risk factors may attribute to unequal power dynamics and may in turn influence an individual's socio-economic position (i.e. economic vulnerability and HIV infection) (UNAIDS, 2016; Mbirimtengerenji, 2007; Mufune, 2014; Rodrigoa & Rajapakseb, 2010). The vulnerability of AGYW is further illustrated through the societal norms of male superiority and poverty, making AGYW unable to negotiate safe sex practices (UNAIDS, 2016; Rodrigoa & Rajapakseb, 2010). The inability to negotiate safe sex practices may subsequently lead to the engagement of risky sexual behaviours (Niëns & Lowery, 2009; Wilson, Wright, Safrit & Rudy, 2010) which contributes toward high HIV infection rates.

A crucial intervention aimed at reducing the HIV infection rate is HIV counselling and testing (HCT). HCT informs individuals of their HIV status and enables HIV positive individuals to receive the necessary care and treatment in order to live a healthy life in spite of living with HIV (Tenkorang & Maticka-Tyndale, 2013). This assists in the reduction of the risk of further HIV transmission and encourages HIV-negative individuals to maintain their status (Peltzer, Matseke, Mzolo & Majaja, 2009). HCT is therefore essential for both knowledge of one's HIV status as well as HIV prevention.

Perception of risk is an important driver of HIV testing. Although not always the case, AGYW in a study by Tenkorang (2016) who perceived themselves as at risk proceeded to getting themselves tested. Thus, adolescents that perceive themselves at risk of contracting HIV may behave in such a way as to reduce their HIV risk. The ways in which AGYW will reduce their risk are through having an HIV test, knowing their HIV status and seeking knowledge about HIV (Sherr et al., 2007; Tenkorang et al., 2009; Tenkorang and Maticka-Tyndale, 2013).

However, a large proportion of new infections are spread through lack of awareness of one's HIV status (Marks, Crepaz & Janssen, 2006). This lack of awareness may in part be due to the fear and beliefs around HCT, which Strauss, Rhodes and George (2015) in turn found could be a result of insufficient knowledge about HCT. Insufficient knowledge may be due to the lack of knowledge of HIV testing (i.e. testing sites) (Choi, Lui, Guo, Han, & Mandel, 2006). Knowledge about HIV and sexual and reproductive health education are preventative measures which may increase the uptake of HIV testing and in turn reduce the risk of HIV (Shisana et al. 2014; UNAIDS 2016; Salam et al., 2016; Simbayi et al., 2019).

Globally, there is a low level (23%) of correct knowledge of HIV among AGYW (UNAIDS, 2019a). Although slightly higher than the global HIV knowledge level, knowledge of HIV levels remains low (31%) among AGYW in sub-Saharan Africa (UNAIDS, 2019a). Low levels of HIV knowledge are a risk as it makes individuals vulnerable and susceptible to HIV infection (Israel, Lauder & Simonetti, 2008). Hence, HIV knowledge is seen as a protective factor against HIV infection as studies reported a positive association between knowledge about HIV and a reduction in risky sexual behaviour (Bertrand et al., 2006).

From several studies, it is evident that there is a gap in HIV knowledge among AGYW. The knowledge gap may be at the uptake of HCT. Although there appears to be low levels of HIV knowledge among AGYW, research is limited. If we know what factors are associated with low HIV knowledge, we might be able to better tailor our interventions. Improved understanding of HIV knowledge will assist in improving ways to prevent and reduce HIV infection among AGYW. Therefore, research ought to address this understudied area with particular focus on knowledge of HIV and its associations with both demographic and behavioural characteristics. In this study, we aimed to investigate knowledge and perceptions about HIV risk behaviours in females aged 15-24 years and to explore any associations with demographic and behavioural characteristics.

Objectives

To examine the demographic and behavioral characteristics that influence knowledge about HIV among AGYW by:

1. Describing knowledge of HIV (transmission and prevention) among young women aged 15 - 24 years enrolled in the SABSSM IV survey.
2. Investigating the association between knowledge of HIV (transmission and prevention) and:

a) Socio-demographic characteristics (age, race, locality, province, education, marital status, employment status))

b) Behavioural characteristics (risk associated –, risk perception, ever had HIV test/ever tested,awareness of HIV status, sexual activity, multiple sexual partners, condom use, alcohol use)

Methods

Study design and sample for the parent study

This was a sub-study based on the 2012 South African National HIV Prevalence, Incidence and Behaviour Survey, a cross-sectional population-based household survey that employed a multistage stratified cluster sampling approach to the select study population.

The parent study systematically selected a random sample of 15 households from each of 1000 enumeration areas (EAs). These were stratified by province, locality and race as defined by the South African national statistical agency, Statistics South Africa (Statistics South Africa, 2013). The questionnaires which were age appropriate consisting of questions pertaining to demographics, HIV-related knowledge, practices, attitudes and behaviours were administered. In addition to this, dry blood spots (DBS) specimens were collected from consenting participants for HIV testing. Ethical approval was obtained from HSRC Research Ethics Committee and by both the CDC Division of Global HIV and TB and the Centre for Global Health prior to its implementation REC number: 5/17/11/10 (see Appendix 1).

Study design and sample for the sub-study

For this study, only the questions on sociodemographic and HIV related behaviours were analysed for AGYW aged 15 - 24 years. The primary outcome measure was knowledge of HIV. Ethical approval was obtained from UCT Ethics Committee and a reciprocal approval obtained from HSRC Research Ethics Committee prior to commencement REC number: 462/2018 (see Appendix 4)

Measures

Demographic characteristics were measured through self-reported age, race, locality, province, education, marital status, employment status (Table 1). Behavioural characteristics were measured through self-reported risk perception, HIV testing, awareness of HIV status, sexual activity, multiple sexual partners, condom use and alcohol use.

Knowledge about HIV (transmission and prevention) was measured using a composite measure of precise knowledge, which was created out of responses to three prompted questions related to HIV transmission and prevention and two myths and misconceptions about the transmission of the disease (Table 2). This study only represents the proportion of respondents that answered both sets of questions correctly. Therefore, knowledge is defined by correctly identifying ways of preventing HIV transmission and rejecting major misconceptions about HIV transmission. Having low levels of HIV knowledge indicate that not all knowledge questions and misconceptions were correctly answered and having high levels of HIV knowledge indicate correct knowledge of both the two prevention questions and rejection of the three misconceptions about HIV.

Statistical analysis

The statistical analysis, which did not take clustering into account, was done on weighted data using STATA software package version 13. To ensure representative data, the final weighted data was benchmarked to the official Statistics South Africa national midyear population estimates by age, race, sex and province. Descriptive statistics by chi-squared analysis was used to demonstrate sociodemographic and behavioural characteristics; while bivariate and multivariate logistic regression was used to determine which variables were associated with HIV knowledge. Only the results that yielded statistical significance by the bivariate analysis were included in the multivariate analysis. A multivariate regression model was fitted to AGYW aged 15-24 years; p values less than 0.05 were considered statistically significant and odds ratios (ORs) with 95% confidence intervals (CI) reported.

Results

Summary of Demographic variables

Of the overall sample size of 3700 used in this study, 51.1% were aged 15-19 years and 48.9% were aged 20-24 years (Table 3). Majority were Black African (83.5%); from an urban formal geotype (48.5%), from KwaZulu-Natal (23.2%), unemployed (87.8%), not married (94.7%) and had completed secondary level education (Table 3).

Associations with HIV Knowledge

<u>Demographics</u>

Overall, AGYW displayed low levels of correct HIV knowledge (29.0%; 95%CI 26.7-31.4) (Table 4); the highest proportion of correct knowledge of HIV was displayed by older

AGYW aged 20-24 years (30.1%) Indians (58.4%), those living in urban formal settings (34.0%), the Free State (37.3%), those who were employed (40.0%), not married (29.5%), and those with tertiary as the highest level of education (44.3%).

Socio-behavioural

Overall, AGYW displayed low levels of correct HIV knowledge. The highest proportion of correct knowledge of HIV was displayed by AGYW who had a high risk perception of getting HIV (30.3%), those who ever tested for HIV (30.4%), those who were aware of their current HIV status (31.1%), those who had sex in the last 12 months (29.7%), those who had multiple sexual partners in the last 12 months (39.6%), those who used a condom at last sex in the last 12 months (30.7%), and those who were high risk alcohol users (43.5%) (Table 5).

Logistic Regression Analysis
Demographics

White AGYW were more likely to have correct HIV knowledge [OR=2.44 (95% CI: 1.48-4.03), p=0.001] compared to Black Africans; Indian AGYW were significantly more likely to have correct HIV knowledge [OR=3.85 (95% CI: 2.39-6.18), p=0.000] compared to Black Africans (Table 6).

AGYW in urban informal settings were significantly less likely to have correct HIV knowledge [OR=0.64 (95% CI: 0.45-0.90), p=0.011] compared to urban formal settings; AGYW in rural informal settings were significantly less likely to have correct HIV knowledge [OR=0.57 (95% CI: 0.33-0.98), p=0.043] compared to urban formal settings (Table 6).

AGYW in Eastern Cape were significantly less likely to have correct HIV knowledge [OR=0.69 (95% CI: 0.48-1.00), p=0.048] compared to Western Cape; AGYW in KwaZulu-Natal were significantly less likely to have correct HIV knowledge [OR=0.69 (95% CI: 0.48-0.99), p=0.044] compared to Western Cape; AGYW in North West were significantly less likely to have correct HIV knowledge [OR=0.50 (95% CI: 0.32-0.77), p=0.002] compared to Western Cape; AGYW in Limpopo were significantly less likely to have correct HIV knowledge [OR=0.44 (95% CI: 0.27-0.71), p=0.001] compared to Western Cape (Table 6).

Socio-behavioural

Socio-economic status

AGYW that were unemployed were significantly less likely to have correct HIV knowledge [OR=0.57 (95% CI: 0.40-0.80), p=0.001] compared to AGYW that were employed (Table 6).

AGYW whose highest level of education was matric were significantly more likely to have correct HIV knowledge [OR=1.66 (95% CI: 1.04-2.64), p=0.034] compared to AGYW that had no or a primary level education; AGYW that highest level of education was tertiary education were significantly more likely to have correct HIV knowledge [OR=2.68 (95% CI: 1.47-4.89), p=0.001] compared to AGYW that had no or a primary level education (Table 6).

Sexual behaviour

AGYW that had sex in the last 12 months were significantly more likely to have correct HIV knowledge [OR=1.70 (95% CI: 1.08-2.72), p=0.023] compared to AGYW that did not have sex in the last 12 months (Table 7).

AGYW that had multiple sexual partners in the last 12 months were significantly less likely to have correct HIV knowledge [OR=0.60 (95% CI: 0.39-0.99), p=0.045] compared to AGYW that had 1 sexual partner in the last 12 months (Table 7).

AGYW with a low risk of alcohol use were significantly more likely to have correct HIV knowledge [OR=1.4 (95% CI: 1.02-1.87), p=0.039] compared to AGYW that abstained from alcohol (Table 7).

Multivariate Regression Analysis

Only those variables that were significantly associated with HIV knowledge were included in the multiple regression model (Table 8). The final model showed that among AGYW, only 1 variable showed significance and that was the urban informal geotype. AGYW in urban informal settings were significantly less likely to have correct HIV knowledge [aOR=0.59 (95% CI: 0.35-0.99), p=0.046] compared to all geotypes. This is indicative that there is an HIV knowledge deficit in urban informal settings.

Discussion

This study found that AGYW in South Africa displayed a low level of HIV knowledge across race, geotype, province and sexual activity. Low levels of HIV knowledge were found, more specifically to be associated with AGYW living in urban informal areas.

Indian AGYW displayed the highest proportion of HIV knowledge. The bivariate analysis also confirmed that Indian as well as White AGYW had higher HIV knowledge compared to Black Africans. This may be because of South Africa's history of Apartheid, which perpetuated race-based inequalities and in turn affected access to sexual and reproductive health (Gilbert & Selikow, 2011).

AGYW from the Free State province displayed the highest proportion of HIV knowledge. The bivariate analysis found that AGYW in Eastern Cape, KwaZulu-Natal, North West, and Limpopo provinces had low HIV knowledge compared to AGYW in Western Cape Province. This may be due to Western Cape having relatively better infrastructure and resources as well as the presence of the Treatment Action Campaign (TAC), which provides the imperative access (through HIV education) to HIV treatment (Grebe, 2011).

AGYW that were employed displayed the highest proportion of HIV knowledge. The bivariate analysis also confirmed that AGYW that were unemployed had low HIV knowledge compared to AGYW that were employed. This could be linked to both the age of the AGYW (i.e. may still be students at some level of education), availability of resources and socioeconomic status (UNAIDS, 2019a).

AGYW with tertiary as the highest level of education displayed the highest proportion of HIV knowledge. The bivariate analysis also confirmed that AGYW that highest level of education was matric and tertiary level had high HIV knowledge compared to AGYW that had no or a primary level education. These findings are in agreement with previous findings which indicated an association between HIV knowledge and level of education (i.e. as level of education increased, so did knowledge of HIV) (South African Demographic and Health survey (Chambers, Haile, Richardson, & Richardson, 2002; Burgoyne & Drummond, 2008).

AGYW that had a high-risk perception of getting HIV displayed the highest proportion of HIV knowledge., The finding is in line with the assumption of adolescents that perceive themselves at risk of contracting HIV will behave in such a way as to reduce their risk. There are a number of ways in which they will reduce their risk, including but not limited to having an HIV test done, knowing their HIV status; being knowledgeable about the disease as well as learning from those infected with HIV (Sherr et al., 2007; Tenkorang et al., 2009; Tenkorang & Maticka-Tyndale, 2013).

AGYW who ever-tested for HIV displayed the highest proportion of HIV knowledge. HIV testing (i.e. ever-tested for HIV) is consistent with research that knowledge about HIV may affect the uptake of HCT (Shisana et al., 2014; UNAIDS, 2016).

AGYW who were aware of their current HIV status displayed the highest proportion of HIV knowledge. Awareness of current HIV status may be due to having sufficient knowledge, access to and knowledge of testing sites.

AGYW who had multiple sexual partners in the last 12 months, who used a condom at last sex in the last 12 months, and who were high-risk alcohol users displayed the highest proportion of HIV knowledge. Bertrand et al. (2006) found that knowledge of HIV transmission positively affects risky sexual behaviours (i.e. multiple sexual partners) such that having HIV knowledge decreases risky sexual behaviour. AGYW with a low risk of alcohol use had low HIV knowledge compared to AGYW that abstained from alcohol. This finding agrees with evidence that low risk alcohol use plays a protective role against HIV infection among AGYW (Kalichman, Simbayi, Kaufma, Cain, Jooste, 2007).

AGYW living in in urban formal settings displayed the highest proportion of HIV knowledge; the bivariate analysis also confirmed that AGYW in urban and rural informal settings had poor HIV knowledge compared to AGYW living in urban formal settings. Furthermore, the regression analysis also confirmed that AGYW living in urban informal settings had low HIV knowledge compared to all geotypes. This is indicative that there is an HIV knowledge deficit in urban informal settings. This may be attributed to the high levels of poverty and inequality in South Africa, which causes an economic and social disadvantage of AGYW to knowledge around HIV transmission (Statistics South Africa, 2020). AGYW in urban informal settings may have unequal access to healthcare, education, employment opportunities because of their low relative socioeconomic status (Lopman, Lewis, Nyamukapa, Mushati, Chandiwana, Gregson; 2007; Shishana et al., 2014; UNAIDS,2019b). Low relative socio-economic status has been found to be associated with HIV risk infection especially among AGYW (Mbirimtengerenji, 2007; Mufune, 2014; Rodrigoa & Rajapakseb, 2010).

We found some variation in HIV knowledge, which we can explain given the existing literature and our understanding of South Africa, but even so, the overall knowledge levels remained quite low, even among those sub-groups with higher knowledge scores. This knowledge deficit may be due to a lack of knowledge dissemination, education and access to sexual and reproductive healthcare facilities.

South Africa's response from 2012-2017 to HIV knowledge with regard to HIV prevention were through social and behaviour change communication programmes (Simbayi et al., 2019). These interventions were made up of nongovernmental organisations such as Soul City, Centre for Communication Impact, loveLife, and Community Media Trust implemented HIV communication programmes. In addition, a campaign called Phila led by the NDoH was initiated in late 2015. HCT were expanded in 2013 to include diverse settings (including farms) getting people to undergo testing (SANAC, 2015). Other initiatives included mobilisation activities in the form of multi-media, school based and the broader community, as well as the provision of HIV information by civil organisation (UNAIDS, 2014, UNAIDS, 2016).

It is clear that these interventions had a positive impact on AGYW with regards to HIV knowledge, as knowledge of HIV transmission showed a slight improvement from 2012 (29.0%) to the 2017 (36.2%) (Simbayi et al., 2019). However, despite this increase, correct HIV knowledge levels among AGYW generally remained low. Thus making this study relevant in a contemporary setting.

Study limitations are that the nature of the study does not allow for causality measures. Therefore, the study was unable to establish causal relationships i.e. what causes low/high levels of HIV knowledge. Most of the variables were self-reported and may have been influenced by social desirability or recall bias. Therefore, a true reflection of the levels of HIV knowledge may be distorted as the relationship/correlation/association found might reflect the response bias instead of a genuine relationship between variables that are being measured. Having excluded other covariates that could have potentially been of relevance to HIV knowledge could have an effect on HIV knowledge that was not found among the covariates studied. The study used multivariate logistic regression to analyse the data, this method does not adjust for correlated observations. This may have led to biased confidence intervals making the study findings less concrete.

Conclusion

This study concludes that AGYW has a lack of knowledge around HIV, which could be attributed to a number of factors. It ought to be addressed through the improvement of existing intervention or the implementation of new interventions aimed at increasing the knowledge of AGYW around HIV. Focus should be on the AGYW living in urban informal settings, as there appears to be a knowledge deficit among AGYW in urban informal settings. Therefore, the main findings emphasise the need to address the structural socio-economic drivers of HIV among AGYW. This ought to be done by targeting those that come from urban informal settings. A critical gap of HIV knowledge has been identified in the prevention cascade. Correct knowledge is needed to ensure that effective prevention strategies are tailored to the needs of this vulnerable population. These needs can be addressed through the promotion of knowledge through education and equitable and accessible availability of education and sexual and reproductive health services and HCT and support among AGYW particularly in the rural and urban informal areas.

Table legend

- Table 1 represents a summary of demographic variables measured in the study
- Table 2 represents a summary of HIV Transmission Knowledge and prevention measures used in the study
- Table 3 represents basic demographic characteristics of the sample.
- Table 4 represents the extent of correct knowledge about HIV transmission and the rejection of the misconceptions about HIV transmission by demographic characteristics of AGYW.
- Table 5 represents the extent of correct knowledge about HIV transmission and the rejection of the misconceptions about HIV transmission by socio-behavioural characteristics of AGYW.
- Table 6 represents the bivariate analysis, which is a bivariate logistic regression of demographic characteristics associated with HIV knowledge.
- Table 7 represents the bivariate analysis, which is a bivariate logistic regression of socio-behavioural characteristics associated with HIV knowledge.
- Table 8 represents the multivariate analysis, which is a multivariate logistic regression of variables associated with HIV knowledge.

References

1. Bertrand, J. B., O'Reilly, K., Denison, J. Anhang, R, Sweat, M. (2006). Systematic review of the effectiveness of mass communication programs to change HIV/AIDS-related behaviors in developing countries, *Health Education Research, 21*, 567–597.

2. Burgoyne, A. D. & Drummond, P. D. (2008). Knowledge of HIV and AIDS in women in sub-Saharan Africa. *African Journal of Reproductive Health, 12,*14-31.

3. Campbell, C. (2019) Social capital, social movements and global public health: fighting for health-enabling contexts in marginalised settings. *Social Science and Medicine.*

4. Celum, C. L., Moretlwe, S. D., McConnell, M, van Rooyen, H., Bekker, L. G., Kurth, A. Bukusi, E., Desmond, C., Morton, J & Baeten, J. M. (2015). Rethinking HIV prevention to prepare for oral PrEP implementation for young African women. *Journal of the International AIDS Society 2015, 18*, 20227.

5. Chambers, J., Haile, B., Richardson, A. richardson, C. (2001). Annual conference HIV?AIDS survey: analyses and implications. Annual Conference of the 19th Episcopal District of the African Methodist Episcopal District of the African Episcopal Church. Johannesburg, South Africa 2002.

6. Choi, K. H., Lui, H., Guo, Y., Han, L., & Mandel, J. S. (2006). Lack of HIV testing and awareness of HIV infection among men who have sex with men, Beijing, China. *AIDS Education and Prevention, 18*, 33-43.

7. Dellar, R.C; Dlamini, S & Karim, Q. A. (2015). Adolescent girls and young women: key populations for HIV epidemic control. *Journal of the International AIDS Society, 18,* 64-70.

8. Doyle, A. M., Mavedzenge, S. N., Plummer, M. L., Ross, D. A. (2012). The sexual behaviour ofadolescents in sub-Saharan Africa: patterns and trends from national surveys. *Tropical Medicine & International Health, 17,* 796–807.

9. DREAMS South Africa fact sheet (2016).

10. Fako, T. T. (2006). Social and psychological factors associated with willingness to test for HIV infection among young people in Botswana. *AIDS Care, 18*, 201–207.

11. Gilbert, L, Selikow T. A. (2011). The epidemic in this country has the face of a woma: gender and HIV/AIDS in South Africa. *Afr J AIDS Res. 10*, 325–34.

12. Global AIDS update 2016: fast-tracking the response in eastern and southern Africa – focus on Adolescent Girls & Young Women. Global AIDS update 2016, and prevention gap report, UNAIDS, Geneva; 2016. Geneva: UNAIDS.

13. Glynn, J. R., Carael, M., Buve, A., Anagonou, S., Zekeng, L., Kahindo, M., et al. (2004). Does increased general schooling protect against HIV infection? A study in four African cities. *Tropical Medicine & International Health, 9*, 4–14.

14. Govender, K., Masebo, W., Nyamaruze, P., Cowden, R. G., Schunter, B. T., & Bains, A. (2018). HIV Prevention in Adolescents and Young People in the Eastern and Southern African Region: A Review of Key Challenges Impeding Actions for an Effective Response. *The open AIDS journal, 12*, 53–67.

15. Grebe, E (2011). The Treatment Action Campaign's Struggle for AIDS Treatment in South Africa. Journal of Southern African Studies, 37:2011.

16. Gregson, S. Terceira, N., Mushati, P., Nyamukapa, C. Campbell, C. (2004). Community group participation: Can it help young women to avoid HIV? An exploratory study of social capital and school education in rural Zimbabwe. *Soc Sci Med, 58*, 2119–2132.

17. Harrison, A., Colvin, C. J, Kuo, C., Swartz, A., & Lurie, M. (2015). Sustained high HIV incidence in young women in southern Africa: social, behavioral and structural factors and emerging intervention approaches. *Current HIV/AIDS Reports, 12*, 207.

18. Israel, E., Laudar, C. & Simonetti, C. (2008). HIV prevention among vulnerable populations: Pathfinder International Technical Guidance Series Number 6.

19. Jewkes, R. K., Dunkle, K., Nduna, M., & Shai, N. (2010). Intimate partner violence, relationship power inequity, and incidence of HIV infection in young women in South Africa: a cohort study. *Lancet, 376,* 41–48.

20. Johnson, L.F, Chiu, C., Myer, L., Davies, M., Dorrington, R.E., Bekker, L., et al. (2016). Prospects for HIV control in South Africa: a model-based analysis. *Global Health Action, 9*, 30314.

21. Jukes M, Simmons S, Bundy D. (2008). Education and vulnerability: the role of schools in protecting young women and girls from HIV in southern Africa. *Aids 22*, 41–56.

22. Kennedy, B. P., Kawachi, I.,Glass, R & Prothrow-Stith, D. 1998. "Income distribution, socioeconomic status and self-rated health in the United States," *Brit. Med. J.* 317: pp. 917-921.

23. Kharsany, A. B. M. & Karim, Q. A. (2016). HIV Infection and AIDS in Sub-Saharan Africa: Current Status, Challenges and Opportunities. *The Open AIDS Journal, 10*, 34-48.

24. Kalichman, S. C., & Simbayi, L. C. (2003). HIV testing attitudes, AIDS stigma, and voluntary HIV Counselling and Testing in a black township in Cape Town, South Africa. *Sexually Transmitted Infections, 79*, 442-447.

25. Kalichman, S. C., Simbayi, L. C., Kaufma, M., Cain, D., & Jooste, S. (2007). Alcohol use and sexual risks for HIV/AIDS in sub-Saharan Africa: systematic review of empirical findings. *Prevention Science, 8*, 141–151.

26. Lopman B, Lewis J, Nyamukapa C, Mushati P, Chandiwana S, Gregson S. (2007). HIV incidence and poverty in Manicaland, Zimbabwe: Is HIV becoming a disease of the poor? *AIDS, 21*, 57-66.

27. MacPhail, C. L., Pettifor, A., Coates T., Rees, H. (2008). 'You must do the test to know your status': attitudes to HIV voluntary counseling and testing for adolescents among South African youth and parents. *Health Education & Behavior, 35*, 87–104.

28. MacPhail, C., Pettifor, A., Moyo, W., Rees, H (2009). Factors associated with HIV testing among sexually active South African youth aged 15–24 years. *AIDS Care, 2*, 41–67.

29. Marks, G., Crepaz, N. & Janssen, R.S. (2006). Estimating sexual transmission of HIV from persons aware and unaware that they are infected with the virus in the USA. *AIDS, 20*,1447–50.

30. Maughan-Brown, B., George, G., Beckett, S., Evans, M., Lewis, L., Cawood, C., Khanyile, D., & Kharsany, A. (2018). HIV Risk Among Adolescent Girls and Young Women in Age-Disparate Partnerships: Evidence From KwaZulu-Natal, South Africa. *Journal of acquired immune deficiency syndromes (1999)*, *78*(2), 155–162.

31. Mbirimtengerenji, N. D. (2007). Is HIV/AIDS Epidemic Outcome Of poverty in sub-Saharan Africa? *Croatian Medical Journal, 48*, 605–17.

32. Mufune, P. (2014). Poverty and HIV/AIDS in Africa: specifying the connections. *Social Theory & Health, 1*, 1–29.

33. Ndifuna Ukwazi Treatment Action Campaign [online] Available at: https://nu.org.za

34. Niëns, L. & Lowery, D. (2009). Gendered epidemiology: sexual equality and the prevalence of HIV/AIDS in sub-Saharan Africa. *Social Science Quarterly,90*, 1134–1144.

35. Njagi, F., & Maharaj, P. (2006). Access to voluntary counselling and testing services: perspectives of young people. *South Africa Review of Sociology, 37*, 113–27.

36. Peltzer, K., Matseke, G., Mzolo, T., & Majaja, M. (2009). Determinants of knowledge of HIV status in South Africa: results from a population-based HIV survey. *BioMedCentral Public Health, 9,* 174.

37. Peltzer, K. & Matseke G. (2013). Determinants of HIV testing among young people aged 18 – 24 years in South Africa. *African Health Science, 13,* 1012-1020.

38. PEPFAR (2017). *Annual report to congress.*

39. Pettifor, A. E., Rees, H. V., Kleinschmidt, I., Steffenson, A. E., MacPhail, C., Hlongwa-Madikizela, L, et al. (2005). Young people's sexual health in South Africa: HIV prevalence and sexual behaviors from a nationally representative household survey. *AIDS, 19,* 1525–1534.

40. Pettifor, A., Stoner, M., Pike, C., & Bekker, L. G. (2018). Adolescent lives matter: preventing HIV in adolescents. *Current opinion in HIV and AIDS, 13*(3), 265–273.

41. Pettifor A, MacPhail C, Rees H & Cohen M. HIV and sexual behavior among young people (2008): the South African paradox. *Sexually Transmitted Diseases, 35,* 843–844.

42. Psaros, C., Milford, C., Smit, J.A., Greener, L., Mosery, N. Matthews, L.T., . . . Safren, S. A. (2018). HIV Prevention among young women in South Africa: Understanding multiple layers of risk. *Archives of Sexual Behaviour, 47,* 1969-1982.

43. Rodrigoa ,C. & Rajapakseb, S. (2010). HIV, poverty and women. International Health, 2, 9–16.

44. SANAC (South African National Aids Council) (2015) A review of the South African comprehensive HIV AIDS grant. Pretoria: Department of Health.

45. SANAC (2018). Adolescent Girls and Young Women (AGYW) Summit. http://sanac.org.za/2018/04/20/adolescent-girls-and-young-women-agyw-summit-24-25-april-2018/

46. Salam, R.A., Faqqah, A, Sajjad, N., Lassi, Z. S. Das, J.K., Kaufman, M. Bhutta, Z.A. (2016). Improving Adolescent Sexual and Reproductive Health: A Systematic Review of Potential Interventions. *Journal of Adolescent Health, 59,* 11- 28.

47. Sherr, L., Lopman B., Kakowa M., Dube S., Chawira G., Nyamukapa C., et al. (2007). Voluntary counseling and testing: uptake, impact on sexual behavior, and HIV in a rural Zimbabwean cohort. *AIDS, 21,* 851–860.

48. Shisana, O, Rehle, T, Simbayi LC, Zuma, K, Jooste, S, Zungu N, Labadarios, D, Onoya, D et al. (2014) *South African National HIV Prevalence, Incidence and Behaviour Survey, 2012.* Cape Town, HSRC Press.

49. Simbayi, L.C., Zuma, K., Zungu, N., Moyo, S., Marinda, E., Jooste, S., Mabaso, M., Ramlagan, S., North, A., van Zyl, J., Mohlabane, N., Dietrich, C., Naidoo, I. and the SABSSMV Team. (2019). South African National HIV Prevalence, Incidence, Behaviour and Communication Survey, 2017. Cape Town: HSRC Press.

50. Stats SA (Statistics South Africa) (2013) Mid-year population estimates.

51. Strauss, M. Rhodes, B. & George, G. (2015). A qualitative analysis of the barriers and facilitators of HIV counselling and testing perceived by adolescents in South Africa. *BMC Health Services Research, 5,* 1-12.

52. Stöckl, H., Kalra, N., Jacobi, J., & Watts, C.(2013). Is early sexual debut a risk factor for HIV infection among women in sub-Saharan Africa? A systematic review. *American Journal of Reproductive Immunology, 69,* 27–40.

53. Stoner, M.C.D., Nguyen, N., Kilburn K, et al. (2019). Age-disparate partnerships and incident HIV infection in adolescent girls and young women in rural South Africa. *AIDS. 33,* 83-91.

54. Steinert, J. I., Cluver, L., Melendez-Torres, G. J. & Romero, R. H. (2016): Relationships between poverty and AIDS Illness in South Africa: an investigation of urban and rural households in KwaZulu-Natal, Global Public Health, DOI: 10.1080/17441692.2016.1187191

55. Szwarcwalda, C. L., Barbosa-Ju´niorb, A., Pascomb, A. R. & de Souza-Ju´niora, P.R. (2005). Knowledge, practices and behaviours related to HIV transmission among the Brazilian population in the 15–54 years age group. *AIDS, 19,* 51–58.

56. Tenkorang, E. Y. & Maticka-Tyndale E. (2013) Individual-and school- level correlates of HIV testing among secondary school students in Kenya. *Studies in Family Planning, 44,* 169–187.

57. Tenkorang, E. Y. (2016). Perceived vulnerability and HIV testing among youth in Cape Town, South Africa. *Health Promotion International, 31,* 270–279.

58. Thomson, K. A., Baeten, J. M., Mugo, N. R., Bekker, L.G. Celum, C. L. & Heffron, R. (2016). Tenofovir-based Oral PrEP Prevents HIV Infection among Women. *Current Opinion in HIV and AIDS, 11,* 18-26.

59. Treatment Action Campaign About the Treatment Action Campaign [Online] Available at: www.tac.org.za

60. UNAIDS (Joint United Nations Programme on HIV/AIDS). 2004. *World AIDS Campaign 2004: Women, Girls, HIV and AIDS,* Strategic Overview and Background Note. February 2004.

61. UNAIDS. (2013). *Global AIDS response progress reporting 2013: construction of core indicators for monitoring the 2011 UN Political Declaration of HIV/AIDS. Geneva*: UNAIDS.

62. UNAIDS (2014) 90–90–90 An ambitious treatment target to help end the AIDS epidemic. Geneva: UNAIDS.

63. UNAIDS. (2015).

64. UNAIDS. *UNAIDS 2016-2021 Strategy*; August 2015.

65. UNAIDS (2016). HIV prevention among adolescent girls and young women: putting HIV intervention among adolescent girls and young women on the fast-track and engaging men and boys. Geneva: UNAIDS.

66. UNAIDS. *Global AIDS Update 2017;* July 2017. UNAIDS. *AIDSinfo website*; accessed July 2017, available at: http://aidsinfo.unaids.org/. UNAIDS. *Core Epidemiology Slides*; June 2017.

67. UNAIDS. *Fact Sheet 2017*; July 2017.

68. UNAIDS. *Core Epidemiology Slides*; June 2017.

69. UNAIDS data, 2019.

70. UNAIDS, 2019 estimates

71. UNICEF, UNAIDS, WHO. 2002. *Young People And HIV/AIDS: Opportunity in Crisis.*Geneva. 2002.

72. UNAIDS, 2019a. Power to the people.

73. UNAIDS, 2019b. A spotlight on adolescent girls and young women.

74. Wilkinson, R. G. 1996. *Unhealthy Societies: The Afflictions of Inequality.* London: Routledge.

75. Wilkinson, R. G. 2000. *Mind the Gap: Hierarchies, Health, and Human Evolution.*

76. London: Weidenfeld and Nicolson.

77. Wilson, C.M., Wright. P. F., Safrit, J.T. & Rudy, B. (2010). Epidemiology of HIV infection and risk in adolescents and youth. *Journal of Acquired Immune Deficiency Syndrome, 54,* S5-S6.

78. World Health Organization. Guidance on pre-exposure oral prophylaxis (PrEP) for serodiscordant couples, men and transgender women who have sex with men at high risk of HIV: Recommendations for use in the context of demonstration projects. Geneva: 2012. http://www.who.int/hiv/pub/guidance_prep/en/).

79. Yaya, S. Bishwajit, G, Danhoundo, G, Shah, V. & Ekholuenetale, M. (2016). Trends and determinants of HIV/AIDS knowledge among women in Bangladesh. *BMC Public Health, 6*, 1-9.

80. Zuma, K., Shisana, O., Rehle, T. M., Simbayi, L.C., Jooste, S., Zungu, N., Labadarios, D., Onoya, D., Evans, M., Moyo, S. & Abdullah, F. (2016). New insights into HIV epidemic in South Africa: key findings from the National HIV Prevalence, Incidence and Behaviour Survey. *African Journal of AIDS Research, 15,* 67-75.

81. Zuma, T., Seeley, J., Sibiya, L. O., Chimbindi, N., Birdthistle, I., Sherr, L., & Shahmanesh, M. (2019). The Changing Landscape of Diverse HIV Treatment and Prevention Interventions: Experiences and Perceptions of Adolescents and Young Adults in Rural KwaZulu-Natal, South Africa. *Frontiers in public health, 7,* 336.

Tables

Table 1: Summary of demographic variables measured in the study

Measures	Description
Demographic	
Age	By age (15-24 years)
Race	By Race (Black African, White, Coloured, Indian/Asian)
Locality	By geotype (urban formal, urban informal, rural informal, rural formal)
Province	By province (Western Cape, Eastern Cape, Northern Cape, Free State, KwaZulu-Natal, North West, Gauteng, Mpumalanga, Limpopo)
Education	Highest level of education completed i.e. no education/primary (no schooling/grader/grade1-7) secondary (grade8-grade11) matric (grade12) and tertiary (post matric studies complete/ incomplete)
Marital Status	Married (married/civil union) or unmarried (going steady/living together, single, divorced, widow)
Employment status	Employed (employed fulltime/part-time, employed in the formal sector, self-employed fulltime/part-time) or unemployed (unemployed-looking/not looking for work, housewife-looking/not looking for work, sick/disabled/unable to work, student/pupil/learner).
Behavioural	
Risk perception	High-risk perception (definitely will get infected/probably will get infected) and low risk perception (definitely will not get infected/probably will not get infected).
Ever Tested/HIV testing	Ever having an HIV test.
Awareness of HIV status	Having gone for an HIV test in the past 12 months and received and know their HIV status
Sexual Activity	Reporting having had sex in the past 12 months.
Multiple sexual partners	Indication of reported total number of sexual partners in the past 12 months.
Condom use	Indication of condom use at last sex in the past 12 months.
Alcohol use	Abstainers, low risk, risky/hazardous, high risk/harmful and high risk.

Table 2: Summary of HIV Transmission Knowledge and prevention measures used

Knowledge of HIV (Transmission and prevention)		
	Measure	Scoring
	A composite measure of precise knowledge was used (see Appendix 5 or https://www.unaids.org/sites/default/files/media_asset/2017-Global-AIDS-Monitoring_en.pdf pg.102).	Correctly identifying ways of preventing HIV transmission and rejecting major misconceptions about HIV transmission.
Preventing HIV transmission	HIV sexual transmission questions were asked namely, "To prevent HIV infection, a condom must be used for every round of sex, "One can reduce the risk of HIV by having fewer sexual partners" and "Can a healthy-looking person have HIV?"	If the set of questions were answered correctly a score of 1 was assigned, and if answered incorrectly a score of 0 was assigned (UNAIDS, 2013).
Rejecting major misconceptions	Misconception questions namely "Can AIDS be cured", "Can a person get HIV by sharing food with someone who is infected" as recommended by UNAIDS (2013),. An additional question was asked "Can HIV be transmitted from a mother to her unborn baby".	If the set of questions were correctly rejected a score of 1 was assigned, and if any was incorrectly rejected a score of 0 was assigned (UNAIDS, 2013).

Table 3: Summary of Basic demographic characteristics

Variable			
	n	%	95% CI
Age			
15-19 years	1899	51.1	[48.6-53.5]
20-24 years	1801	48.9	[46.5-51.4]
Race			
Black African	2481	83.5	[80.7-85.9]
White	181	5.9	[4.5-7.7]
Coloured	678	8.5	[7.0-10.3]

	n	%	95% CI
Indian/Asian	356	2.1	[1.4-3.3]
Geotype			
Urban formal	2003	48.5	[43.1-53.9]
Urban informal	433	7.1	[5.3-9.4]
Rural informal	989	40.7	[35.4-46.2]
Rural formal	275	3.7	[2.6-5.2]
Province			
Western Cape	419	10.9	[8.7-13.5]
Eastern Cape	479	11.9	[9.3-15.2]
Northern Cape	270	2.2	[1.6-3.0]
Free State	259	5.1	[3.8-6.8]
KwaZulu-Natal	919	23.2	[18.7-28.3]
North West	257	6.4	[5.1-8.0]
Gauteng	462	21.9	[18.0-26.4]
Mpumalanga	282	7.7	[6.0-9.8]
Limpopo	353	10.8	[8.7-13.4]
Employment Status			
Employed	484	12.2	[9.9-14.8]
Unemployed	3068	87.8	[85.2-90.1]
Marital status			
Married	178	5.3	[4.0-6.9]
Not Married	3432	94.7	[93.1-96.0]
Education			
No education/Primary	274	7.8	[6.5-9.3]
Secondary	1872	56.0	[53.2-58.7]
Matric	1005	30.8	[28.0-33.7]
Tertiary	178	5.4	[4.2-7.0]
Total	3700	100.0	

Table 4: Summary statistics of Demographic characteristics by HIV Knowledge

Variable			
	n	%	95% CI
Age			
15-19 years	1899	28.0	[24.9-31.2]
20-24 years	1801	30.1	[27.0-33.4]
Race			

Black African	2481	26.7	[24.3-29.3]
White	181	47.1	[35.4-59.1]
Coloured	678	31.4	[25.7-37.8]
Indian/Asian	356	58.4	[47.0-68.9]
Geotype			
Urban formal	2003	34.0	[30.4-37.7]
urban informal	433	24.6	[19.4-30.8]
Rural informal	989	24.4	[21.1-28.1]
Rural formal	275	22.7	[14.8-33.0]
Province			
Western Cape	419	35.8	[29.7-42.2]
Eastern Cape	479	27.8	[23.1-32.9]
Northern Cape	270	26.6	[18.1-37.2]
Free State	259	37.3	[26.8-49.2]
KwaZulu-Natal	919	27.6	[23.0-32.8]
North West	257	21.7	[16.5-28.0]
Gauteng	462	33.5	[27.8-39.8]
Mpumalanga	282	27.1	[19.3-36.7]
Limpopo	353	19.6	[14.0-26.6]
Employment Status			
Employed	484	40.0	[32.6-48.0]
Unemployed	3068	27.5	[25.2-29.9]
Marital status			
Married	178	25.5	[16.1-37.9]
Not Married	3432	29.5	[27.1-32.0]
Education			
No education/Primary	274	22.9	[16.3-31.1]
Secondary	1872	25.7	[22.8-28.9]
Matric	1005	32.9	[28.5-37.7]
Tertiary	178	44.3	[33.8-55.2]
Total	3700	29.0	[26.7-31.4]

Table 5: Summary statistics of Socio-behavioural characteristics by HIV Knowledge

Variable	n	%	95% CI
Perceived Risk of getting HIV			
High Risk Perception	2971	30.3	[27.7-33.2]
Low Risk Perception	686	24.8	[20.3-30.0]
Ever had an HIV test			
Yes	2127	30.4	[27.8-33.2]
No	1541	26.9	[23.2-30.9]
Aware of HIV current HIV status			
Yes	1581	31.1	[27.7-34.7]
No	2055	27.4	[24.3-30.7]
Had sex in the last 12 months			
No	353	19.8	[13.7-27.7]
Yes	1772	29.7	[26.6-33.0]
Number of sexual partners in the last 12 months			
2+ partners	147	39.6	[29.3-50.9]
1 partner	1619	29.0	[25.9-32.3]
Condom use at last sex in last 12 months			
No	889	29.7	[25.0-34.8]
Yes	844	30.7	[26.3-35.6]
Alcohol use			
Abstainers	2467	27.0	[24.3-29.8]
Low risk (1-7)	648	33.7	[28.1-39.9]
Risky/hazardous level (8-15)	138	37.5	[21.8-56.3]
High risk/harmful (16-19)	30	43.5	[17.4-73.7]
High risk (20+)	15	16.4	[4.6-44.6]

Table 6: Bivariate Logistic Regression of demographic characteristics associated with HIV Knowledge

	Odds Ratio	95% CI		p-value
Age				
15-19	Ref			
20-24	1.11	0.90	1.37	0.334
Race				
Black African	Ref			
White	2.44	1.48	4.03	**0.001**
Coloured	1.26	0.92	1.71	0.146
Indian	3.85	2.39	6.18	**0.000**
Geotype				
Urban formal	Ref			
Urban informal	0.64	0.45	0.90	**0.011**
Rural informal	0.63	0.49	0.81	**0.000**
Rural informal	0.57	0.33	0.98	**0.043**
Province				
Western Cape	Ref			
Eastern Cape	0.69	0.48	1.00	**0.048**
Northern Cape	0.65	0.37	1.14	0.135
Free State	1.07	0.61	1.87	0.810
KwaZulu-Natal	0.69	0.48	0.99	**0.044**
North West	0.50	0.32	0.77	**0.002**
Gauteng	0.91	0.62	1.33	0.617
Mpumalanga	0.67	0.40	1.13	0.131
Limpopo	0.44	0.27	0.71	**0.001**
Employment status				
Employed	Ref			
Unemployed	0.57	0.40	0.80	**0.001**
Marital status				
Married	Ref			
Not married	1.22	0.68	2.22	0.504

Education				
No education/Primary	Ref			
Secondary	1.17	0.74	1.83	0.502
Matric	1.66	1.04	2.64	0.034
Tertiary	2.68	1.47	4.89	**0.001**

Table 7: Bivariate Logistic Regression of socio-behavioural characteristics associated with HIV knowledge

	Odds Ratio	95% CI		p-value
Perceived Risk of getting HIV				
High	Ref			
Low	0.8	0.56	1.02	0.068
Ever had an HIV test				
yes	Ref			
no	0.8	0.67	1.05	0.121
Aware of current HIV status				
Yes	Ref			
No	0.8	0.66	1.05	0.128
Had sex in the last 12 months				
No	Ref			
Yes	1.7	1.08	2.72	**0.023**
Number of sexual partners in the last 12 months				
2+ partners	Ref			
1 partner	0.6	0.39	0.99	**0.045**
Condom use at last sex in last 12 months				
no	Ref			

yes	1.1	0.75	1.47	0.290
Alcohol use				
Abstainers	Ref			
Low risk (1-7)	1.4	1.02	1.87	**0.039**
Risky/hazardous level (8-15)	1.6	0.74	3.57	0.227
High risk/harmful (16-19)	2.1	0.57	7.60	0.265
High risk (20+)	0.5	0.13	2.20	0.385

Table 8: Multiple Regression of variables associated with HIV knowledge

Variable	Odds Ratio	95% CI		p-value
Race				
White	0.73	0.30	1.78	0.492
Coloured	1.40	0.80	2.44	0.227
Indian	0.87	0.38	1.98	0.735
Geotype				
Urban informal	0.59	0.35	0.99	**0.046**
Rural informal	0.71	0.44	1.13	0.152
Rural informal	0.63	0.34	1.14	0.128
Province				
Eastern Cape	1.25	0.63	2.48	0.528
Northern Cape	0.73	0.33	1.61	0.432
Free State	2.12	0.99	4.50	0.050
KwaZulu-Natal	1.32	0.69	2.55	0.400
North West	0.66	0.30	1.42	0.282
Gauteng	0.97	0.50	1.87	0.926
Mpumalanga	0.71	0.30	1.70	0.447
Limpopo	0.83	0.35	1.95	0.669
Employment status				
Unemployed	0.69	0.39	1.21	0.196
Education				
No education/Primary	0.99	0.49	2.04	0.995

Secondary	1.13	0.56	2.26	0.729
Matric	1.31	0.57	3.00	0.519
Tertiary	0.63	0.35	1.15	0.133
Had sex in the last 12 months				
Sex last 12 months (yes)	1.00			
Alcohol use				
Alcohol use-Low risk (1-7)	1.32	0.79	2.21	0.281
Alcohol use-Risky/hazardous level (8-15)	1.14	0.44	3.00	0.784
Alcohol use-High risk/harmful (16-19)	0.24	0.03	1.87	0.174
Alcohol use-High risk (20+)	0.56	0.12	2.62	0.463

Appendices

Appendix 1: Ethical approval

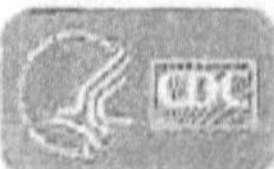

Request for Project Determination & Approval – Center for Global Health (CGH)

This form should be used to submit proposals to the CGH Office of the Associate Director for Science/Laboratory Science (ADS/ADLS) for research/nonresearch determination and requirements for IRB review/approval.

☑ New Request	☐ Amendment	☐ Laboratory Submission

Project Title: 4th South African National HIV, Behavior, and Health Survey, 2011	Project Location/Country(ies): South Africa

Principal Investigator(s):

Project Officer(s): Katherine Robinson, MPH	Division: DGHA	Telephone: +27 12 424 9000 x9012

Proposed Project Dates: Start: 05/01/2011	End: 04/30/2013

Please check appropriate category and subcategory:

☐ **I. Activity is NOT human subjects research. Primary intent is public health practice or a disease control activity (Check one)**
  - ☐ A. Epidemic or endemic disease control activity; Epi-AID # if applicable
  - ☐ B. Routine surveillance activity (e.g., disease, adverse events, injuries)
  - ☐ C. Program evaluation activity
  - ☐ D. Public health program activity*
  - ☐ E. Laboratory proficiency testing

*e.g., service delivery; health education programs; social marketing campaigns; program monitoring; electronic database construction and/or support; development of patient registries; needs assessments; and demonstration projects intended to assess organizational needs, management, and human resource requirements for implementation.

☐ **II. Activity is research but does NOT involve human subjects (Check one)**
  - ☐ A. Activity is research involving collection or analysis of data about health facilities or other organizations or units (NOT persons).
  - ☐ B. Activity is research involving data or specimens from deceased persons.
  - ☐ C. Activity is research involving unlinked or anonymous data or specimens collected for another purpose.
  - ☐ D. Activity is research involving linked data, but CDC non-disclosure form 0.1375B is signed.*
  - ☐ E. Activity is research involving data or specimens from animal subjects.**

*CDC investigators and the holder of the key linking the data to identifiable human subjects enter into an agreement prohibiting the release of the key to the investigators under any circumstances.
**Note: Approval by CDC Institutional Animal Care and Use Committee (IACUC) may be required.

☑ **III. Activity is research involving human subjects but CDC involvement does not constitute "engagement in human subject research" (Check one)**
  - ☑ A. This project is funded under a grant/cooperative agreement/contract award mechanism. Award # U2G PS 000570-01/02/03/04/05
    ALL of the following 3 elements are required:
    - ☑ 1. CDC employees or agents will not intervene or interact with living individuals for research purposes.
    - ☑ 2. CDC employees or agents will not obtain individually identifiable private information.
    - ☑ 3. Supported institution must have a Federalwide Assurance (FWA) and project must be reviewed by a registered IRB linked to the supported institution's FWA.
      Supported Institution/Entity Name: Human Sciences Research Council
      Supported Institution/Entity FWA #: 00006347   FWA Expiration Date (mm/dd/yyyy): 12/10/2012
      Expiration Date of IRB approval: 02/29/2012   (Attach copy of the IRB approval letter)
  - ☐ B. CDC staff provide technical support that does not involve possession or analysis of identifiable data or interaction with participants from whom data are being collected (No current CDC funding).
  - ☐ C. CDC staff are involved only in manuscript writing for a project that has closed. For the project, CDC staff did not interact with participants and were not involved with data collection (No current CDC funding).

Note: Under this category, CDC employee may not interact with human subjects or have access to identifiable data for research purposes. Use of CDC form 0.1375B (referenced above) is also appropriate for additional assurance.

☐ **IV. Activity is research involving human subjects that requires submission to CDC Human Research Protection Office (Check one)***
  - ☐ A. Full Board Review (Use forms 0.1250, 0.1379-signatures, 0.1370-research partners)
  - ☐ B. Expedited Review (Use same forms as A above)
  - ☐ C. Exemption Request** (Use forms 0.1250X, 0.1379-Signatures, 0.1370-research partners)
  - ☐ D. Reliance**
    - ☐ 1. Request to allow CDC to rely on a non-CDC IRB (Use same form as A above, plus 0.1371)
    - ☐ 2. Request to allow outside institution to rely on CDC IRB (Use same forms as A above, plus 0.1372)

*There are other types of requests not listed under category IV, e.g., continuation of existing protocol, amendment, incident reports.
**Exemption and reliance request is approved by CDC Human Research Protection Office (HRPO).

CGH HSR Tracking #:

Amendment: If this request is an amendment to an existing project determination. Please include a brief description of the substantive change or modification below and attach both clean and marked copies of the amended protocol or project outline.

Submission: Attach a protocol or project description (See standard format below) in enough detail to justify the proposed category. Submit your request to your branch chief (or country director for DGHA country staff).

Approval Chain

Investigator → Branch Chief/Country Director → Division ADS → CGH Human Subjects Mailbox

---

CGH ADS/ADLS Review   Date received in CGH ADS /ADLS office: 04/13/2011

[X] Project does not require human subject research review beyond CGH at this time

[ ] Project constitutes human subject research that must be routed to CDC HRPO.

Comments/Rationale for Determination:

Project is approved as category IIIA: activity is human subjects research, but CDC involvement does not constitute engagement in human subjects research. Under this determination, CDC investigators are not permitted to interact with participants or have access to identifiable or linked data for research purposes.

Approvals/Signatures:	Date:	Remarks:
Investigator		on file
Branch Chief/Country Director		on file
Division Human Research Protection Coordinator Division ADS/ADLS or Director	4-13-11	
Human Research Protection Coordinator ADS/ADLS or Deputy ADS/ADLS	04/15/2011	

Note: Although CDC IRB review is not required for certain projects (categories I,II & III) approved under this determination, CDC investigators and project officers are expected to adhere to the highest ethical standards of conduct and to respect and protect to the extent possible the privacy, confidentiality, and autonomy of participants. All applicable country, state, and federal laws must be followed. Informed consent may be appropriate and should address all applicable elements of informed consent. CDC investigators should incorporate diverse perspectives that respect the values, beliefs, and cultures of the people in the country, state, and community in which they work.

Definitions

Agent – A nonemployee of CDC who conducts research under CDC's FWA. This generally includes all persons cleared for access to CDC networks and who use CDC networks or physical facilities for human research activities.

Emergency response – A public health activity undertaken in an urgent or emergency situation, usually because of an identified or suspected imminent health threat to the population, but sometimes because the public and/or government authorities perceive an imminent threat that demands immediate action. The primary purpose of the activity is to document the existence and magnitude of a public health problem in the community and to implement appropriate measures to address the problem (Langmuir, Public Health Reports 1980; 95:470-7).

Engagement – An institution becomes engaged in human subjects research when its employees or agents (i) obtain data about living individuals through intervention or interaction with them for research purposes; (ii) obtain individually identifiable private information about living individuals for research purposes; or (iii) obtain the informed consent of human subjects (http://www.hhs.gov/ohrp TW/Afaq.html). Furthermore, an institution is automatically considered to be engaged in human subjects research whenever it receives a direct HHS award to support such research, even where all activities involving human subjects are carried out by a subcontractor or collaborator.

Human subject or participant – is defined as a living person about whom an investigator conducting research obtains (1) data through intervention or interaction with the individual, or (2) identifiable private information (e.g., medical records, employment records, or school records).

Private information includes information about behavior that occurs in a context in which an individual can reasonably expect that no observation or recording is taking place, and information which has been provided for specific purposes by an individual and which the individual can reasonably expect will not be made public (for example, a medical record). Private information must be individually identifiable (i.e., the identity of the subject is or may readily be ascertained by the investigator or associated with the information) in order for obtaining the information to constitute research involving human subjects.

Program evaluation is the systematic collection of information about the activities, characteristics, and outcomes of programs to make judgments about the program, improve program effectiveness, and/or inform decisions about future program development. Program evaluation should not be confused with treatment efficacy which measures how well a treatment achieves its goals which can be considered as research. CDC guidance on research/non-research

Research – is defined as a systematic investigation, including research development, testing and evaluation, designed to develop or contribute to generalizable knowledge. Activities which meet this definition constitute research, whether or not these activities are conducted or supported under a program which is considered research for other purposes. For example, some demonstration and service programs may include research activities.

Surveillance – The ongoing systematic collection, analysis and interpretation of health data, essential to the planning, implementation and evaluation of public health practice, closely integrated to the dissemination of these data to those who need to know and linked to prevention and control.

Links

- CDC Human Research Protections Policy (2010): http://aops-mas-iis.cdc.gov/Policy/Doc/policy556.pdf
- CDC Distinguishing Public Health Research and Public Health Nonresearch (2010): http://aops-mas-iis.cdc.gov/policy/Doc/policy557.pdf
- HHS Title 45 Code of Federal Regulations Part 46, Protection of Human Subjects (Revised 2009): http://www.cdc.gov/od/science/regs/hrpp/researchDefinition.htm
- OHRP Guidance on Engagement of Institutions in Human Subjects Research: http://www.hhs.gov/ohrp/humansubjects/guidance/engage08.html
- OHRP Guidance on Research Involving Coded Private Information or Biological Specimens: http://www.hhs.gov/ohrp/humansubjects/guidance/cdebiol.htm

NOTE: This page is an outline for a proposal to ensure all required information is included for review and approval. You may submit a proposal following the outline provided below, or a full protocol that includes information pertaining to all applicable elements.

I.   Project Overview
- Project title
- Investigator(s) and roles
- Collaborator(s) and roles, funding mechanism, FWA# (if engaged in research)
- Other participants in research
- Sponsoring institution(s)

II.   Introduction
- Background & Literature review
- Justification for study
- Intended/potential use of study findings
- Design/locations
- Goals and objectives
- Hypotheses or questions
- General approach

III.   Procedures / Methods
- Design
  (How address hypotheses, stakeholder participation, cost benefit, timeline, expedited review requested)
- Study Population
  (Source, case definition, inclusion/exclusion criteria, sampling, enrollment, consent process)
- Variables / Interventions
  (Variables, study instruments, IND/IDE, intervention or treatment, outcomes, training for study personnel)
- Data handling and Analysis
  (Data collection, analysis plan, software, data entry, handling, measurement and tests, potential bias, limitations)
- Handling of Unexpected or Adverse Events
- Dissemination, Notification, and Reporting of Results

IV.   Ethical considerations
- Informed consent
- Confidentiality/privacy protections
- Autonomy
- Additional safeguard for vulnerable populations
- Culture, values, and beliefs

V.   References

VI.   Appendix Materials (data collection forms, consent scripts, scientific peer review, other relevant documents)

A detailed protocol development guide is available at

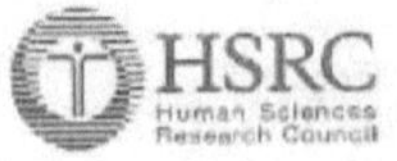

HSRC
Human Sciences
Research Council

Human Sciences Research Council
Lekgotla la Dinyakisišo tša Semahlale tša Setho
Raad vir Geesteswetenskaplike Navorsing
Umkhandlu Wezokucwaninga Ngesayensi Yesintu
Ibhunga Lophando Ngobuzulu-Lwazi Kantu

HSRC Research Ethics Committee
FWA Registration: Organisation No. 0000 6347
IRB No. 00003962
NHREC No.   REC-290808-013

RESEARCH ETHICS COMMITTEE ADMINISTRATION

Room 1411 - HSRC Building
134 Pretorius Street, Pretoria
Gauteng, South Africa
Tel: 27 12 3022009 - Fax: 27 12 3022005
Email: jebotha@hsrc.ac.za - Website: www.hsrc.ac.za
REC tollfree no 0800 212 123

16 February 2011

Prof Leickness Simbayi
HIV/AIDS, STIs & TB (HAST)
Human Sciences Research Council

Dear Prof Simbayi

Amendment to Protocol REC: 5/17/11/10: The Fourth South African National HIV, Behaviour and Health Survey, 2011 (SABSSM IV)

Thank you for your application for ethics approval of an amendment to the above study. This was considered by the Research Ethics Committee at its meeting on 16 February 2011. Ethics Clearance of the amendment to the study was granted.

Principal investigator: Prof Leickness Simbayi

Organisation: Human Sciences Research Council

FWA number: 0000 6347

IRB number: 0000 3962

Cooperative Agreement name: "Improve Capacity of an Indigenous Institute to Enhance M&E of HIV/AIDS in South Africa"

Cooperative Agreement number: 5-U2G-PS00570-04 and 5-U2G-PS00570-05

Protocol title: The Fourth South African National HIV, Behaviour and Health Survey, 2011 (SABSSM IV)

Protocol version: 4.0

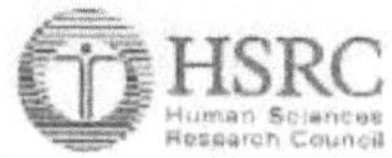

HSRC
Human Sciences
Research Council

Human Sciences Research Council
Lekgotla la Dinyakisišo tša Semahlale tša Setho
Raad vir Geesteswetenskaplike Navorsing
Umkhandlu Wezokucwaninga Ngesigetzi Yesintu
Ibhunga Lophande Ngezuzu-Lwazi Kantu

HSRC Research Ethics Committee
FWA Registration: Organisation No. 0000 6347
IRB No. 00003962
NHREC No.   REC-290808-015

Additional materials reviewed and approved by the REC:

Information Sheet and Consent forms:

a. 18 years and older

b. Head of Household

Information Sheet and Assent forms:

a. Children aged 12 to 17 years of age

b. Children aged 7 to 11 years of age

c. Parent/guardian of children aged 0-17 years

Questionnaires:

a. 15 years and older

b. 12 to 14 year olds

c. Parents/guardians of children younger than 12 years

d. Visiting Point

Protocol date: 21 January 2011

Protocol approval date: 16 February 2011

Date of expiry of protocol approval: 29 February 2012

The Committee wishes you success in your research.

Yours sincerely,

Prof. D R Wassenaar PhD
Chairperson: HSRC REC

Pretoria Office
Room 1411, 134 Pretorius Street, Pretoria, 0002, South Africa. Private Bag X41, Pretoria, 0001,
South Africa. Tel: +27 12 302 2800 Fax: +27 12 302 2828

Cape Town Office
Plein Park Building, 69-83 Plein Street, Cape Town, 8001, South Africa.
Private Bag X9182, Cape Town, 8000, South Africa. Tel: +27 21 466 8000 Fax: +27 21 466 8001

Durban Office
750 Francois Road, Intuthuko Junction, Cato Manor, Durban, 4001, South Africa.
Private Bag X07, Dalbridge, 4014, South Africa. Tel: +27 31 242 5400 Fax: +27 31 242 5401

www.hsrc.ac.za

Appendix 2: Consent forms

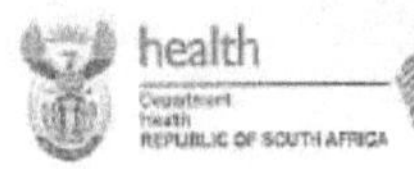 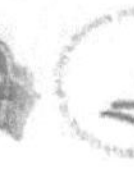 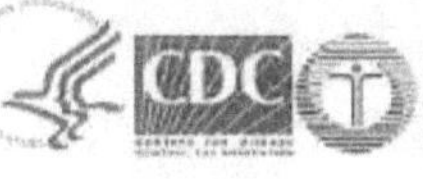 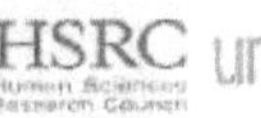 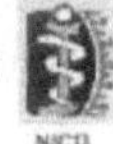 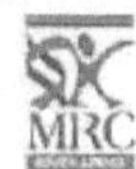

THE FOURTH SOUTH AFRICAN NATIONAL HIV, BEHAVIOUR AND HEALTH SURVEY, 2011/12

Information sheet and Assent form
Participants aged 12 - 17 years old

Introduction

Hello. My name is .... I would like to inform you of a very important scientific study. The study is being done by a group of research organisations led by the Human Sciences Research Council (HSRC) in South Africa and the Centers for Disease Control and Prevention (CDC) in the USA.

Purpose of the study

We are asking all the people aged 12 years and older in the household to respond to some questions. We hope that after combining all people's answers we will learn more about people's health status, and it will assist us with developing effective strategies to improve the health of people living in South Africa.

Please understand that your participation is voluntary. You are not being forced to take part in this study. The choice whether to participate or not is yours alone. However, we would really appreciate it if you do share your thoughts with us. If you choose not take part in answering the questions, you or your household will not be affected in any way. If you agree to participate you may stop me and tell me that you don't want to go on with the interview at any time without any consequences to you or your household.

The information you provide will remain confidential and there will be no "come-backs" from the answers you give me. The information you provide will not in any way be shared with members of your household. I will not be recording your name anywhere on the questionnaire and no one will be able to link you to the answers you give me. Only the researchers will have access to the unlinked information. Any reports or publications that may be written on the findings of the study will be done anonymously.

How long will you need me?

Although your head of household/parent has given us permission to collect information from all members of this household, we also need your permission to take part in the study. If you do agree to participate in the study, your interview by our fieldworker will take between 45 and 90 minutes to complete.

Are there any risks to me if I decide to be in this study?

I will be asking you questions and I ask that you are as open as possible in answering the questions. Some questions may be of a personal and/or sensitive nature and you are free not to answer them if you do not wish to do so. We know that you cannot be absolutely certain about the answers to some of the questions. When it comes to answering questions there are no right and wrong answers.

If I ask you a question which makes you feel sad or upset, we can stop and talk about it. There are also people from ....*(this will be adapted based on organizations operating in the area.)* who have said they are happy to talk with you about those things that upset you, if you need any assistance later. If during the interview we find anything of concern regarding your or your household members, we will refer you or your household member to the nearest clinic for further attention.

What would I have to do if I decide to be in this study?

After the interview you will be asked by a data collector to allow him/her to take a few drops of blood from a finger prick on a special filter paper. Collecting the samples will take about 10 minutes. The drops of blood will be dried on the filter paper which will be then be sent to a laboratory to test for HIV antibodies. If you or someone within the household is interested in knowing the result of your/their HIV test, we will provide you or them with a HIV Specimen Result Request Voucher referring them to a nearby HIV Counseling and Testing site. This voucher will have a unique participant questionnaire number that will assist clinic staff to correctly link the HIV laboratory results to the voucher. Additional information captured on the voucher will include the sex and age of the participant, date of result collection, and the name and address of selected clinic. The clinic staff is aware of the study and will gladly assist you or someone within the household. All that needs to be done is to present the voucher at the clinic. When providing blood samples, please remember that you will also need to give permission to use the blood sample for the current and any ongoing research in the future..

Who should I call if I have questions about this?

This research has been approved by the HSRC Research Ethics Committee (REC). If you any complaints about ethical aspects of the research or feel that you have been harmed in any way by participating in this study, please call the HSRC's toll free ethics hotline 0800 212 123 or the REC Administrator, Khutso Sithole on 012 302 2006. Alternatively, you may send an e-mail to c@tip-offs.com or to to ksithole@hsrc.ac.za . Please note that you do not have to give your name if you do not want to.

If you have concerns or questions about the research you may call the project leaders Mr Sean Jooste at 021 466 7942 or Ms Ntombizodwa Mbelle at 012 302 2614.

Your contribution to this important study is highly valued.

Thank you for your time.

Yours sincerely

Dr. Olive Shisana
Overall Principal Investigator
CEO
HSRC
Cape Town
Tel: (021) 466 8000
Fax: (021) 461 0299

CONSENT

I hereby agree to participate in the South African National HIV, Behaviour and Health survey. I understand that I am participating voluntarily and without being forced in any way to do so. I also understand that I can stop this interview at any point during the interview should I not want to continue and that this decision will not in any way affect me or my household negatively.

I understand that this is a research project the purpose of which is not necessarily to benefit me personally.

I have received the telephone number of a person to contact should I need to report any issues which may arise in this interview.

I understand that this consent form will not be linked to the questionnaire, and that my answers will remain anonumous and confidential.

....
Signature of participant   ....
Date

CONSENT TO PROVIDE A BLOOD SPECIMEN

I hereby agree to provide a finger prick blood specimen as part of the South African National HIV, Behaviour and Health survey. I understand that I am providing the blood specimen voluntarily and without being forced in any way to do so. I also understand that I do not have to provide a blood specimen if I do not want to and that I can stop this interview at any point should I not want to continue, and that this decision will not in any way affect me or my household negatively.

....
Signature of participant   ....
Date

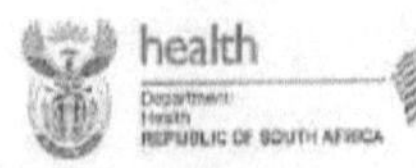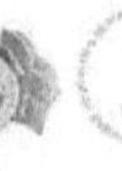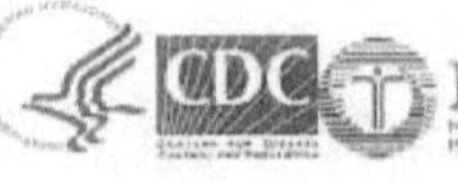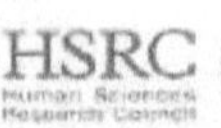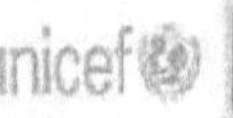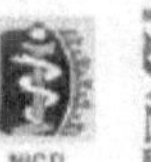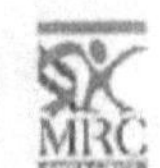

THE FOURTH SOUTH AFRICAN NATIONAL HIV, BEHAVIOUR AND HEALTH SURVEY, 2011/12

Information sheet and Consent form
Participants aged 18 years and older

Introduction

Hello. My name is .... I would like to inform you of a very important scientific study. The study is being done by a group of research organisations led by the Human Sciences Research Council (HSRC) in South Africa and the Centres for Disease Control and Prevention (CDC) in the USA.

What is the purpose of this study?

We are asking all the people aged 12 years and older in the household to respond to some questions. We hope that after combining all people's answers we will learn more about people's health status, and it will assist us with developing effective strategies to improve the health of people living in South Africa.

Please understand that your participation is voluntary. You are not being forced to take part in this study., The choice whether to participate or not is yours alone. However, we would really appreciate it if you do share your thoughts with us. If you choose not take part in answering the questions, you or your household will not be affected in any way. If you agree to participate you may stop me and tell me that you don't want to go on with the interview at any time without any consequences to you or your household.

The information you provide will remain confidential and there will be no "come-backs" from the answers you give me. The information you provide will not in any way be shared with members of your household. I will not be recording your name anywhere on the questionnaire and no one will be able to link you to the answers you give me. Only the researchers will have access to the linked information. Any reports or publications that may be written on the findings of the study will be done anonymously.

How long will you need me?

Although your head of household/parent has given us permission to collect information from all members of this household, we also need your own permission to take part in the study. Your interview by our fieldworker will take between 45 and 90 minutes to complete.

Are there any risks to me if I decide to be in this study?

I will be asking you questions and I ask that you are as open as possible in answering the questions. Some questions may be of a personal and/or sensitive nature and you are free not to answer them if you do not wish to do so. We know that you cannot be absolutely certain about the answers to some of the questions. When it comes to answering questions there are no right and wrong answers.

If I ask you a question which makes you feel sad or upset, we can stop and talk about it. There are also people from ....(*this will be adapted based on organizations operating in the area.*) who have said they are happy to talk with you about those things that upset you, if you need any assistance later. If during the interview we find anything of concern regarding your or your household members, we will refer you or your household member to the nearest clinic for further attention.

What would I have to do if I decide to be in this study?

After the interview you will be asked by a data collector to allow him/her to take a few drops of blood from a finger prick on a special filter paper. Collecting the samples will take about 10 minutes. The drops of blood will be dried on the filter paper which will be then be sent to a laboratory to test for HIV antibodies. If you are interested in knowing the result of your HIV test, we will provide you with a HIV Specimen Result Request Voucher referring them to a nearby HIV Counseling and Testing site. This voucher will have a unique participant questionnaire number that will assist clinic staff to correctly link the HIV laboratory results to the voucher. Additional information captured on the voucher will include the sex and age of the participant, date of result collection, and the name and address of selected clinic. The clinic staff is aware of the study and will gladly assist you. All that needs to be done is to present the voucher at the clinic. When providing blood samples, please remember that you will also need to give permission to use the blood sample for the current and any ongoing research in the future.

Who should I call if I have questions about this?

This research has been approved by the HSRC Research Ethics Committee (REC). If you any complaints about ethical aspects of the research or feel that you have been harmed in any way by participating in this study, please call the HSRC's toll free ethics hotline 0800 212 123 or the REC Administrator, Khutso Sithole on 012 302 2006. Alternatively, you may send an e-mail to c@tip-offs.com or to to ksithole@hsrc.ac.za . Please note that you do not have to give your name if you do not want to.

If you have concerns or questions about the research you may call the project leaders Mr Sean Jooste at 021 466 7942 or Ms Ntombizodwa Mbelle at 012 302 2614.

Your contribution to this important study is highly valued.

Thank you for your time.

Yours sincerely

Dr. Olive Shisana
Overall Principal Investigator
CEO
HSRC
Cape Town
Tel: (021) 466 8000
Fax: (021) 461 0299

CONSENT

I hereby agree to participate in the South African National HIV, Behaviour and Health survey. I understand that I am participating voluntarily and without being forced in any way to do so. I also understand that I can stop this interview at any point during the interview should I not want to continue and that this decision will not in any way affect me or my household negatively.

I understand that this is a research project the purpose of which is not necessarily to benefit me personally.

I have received the telephone number of a person to contact should I need to report any issues which may arise in this interview.

I understand that this consent form will not be linked to the questionnaire, and that my answers will remain anonymous and confidential.

....

Signature of participant   **Date**

CONSENT TO PROVIDE A BLOOD SPECIMEN

I hereby agree to provide a finger prick blood specimen as part of the South African National HIV, Behaviour and Health survey. I understand that I am providing the blood specimen voluntarily and without being forced in any way to do so. I also understand that I do not have to provide a blood specimen if I do not want to and that I can stop this interview at any point should I not want to continue, and that this decision will not in any way affect me or my household negatively.

....

Signature of participant   **Date**

Appendix 3: Questionnaire

Appendix 3: Questionnaire

Questionnaire number:

Barcode

YOUTH AND ADULT: PERSONS 15 YEARS OLD AND OLDER

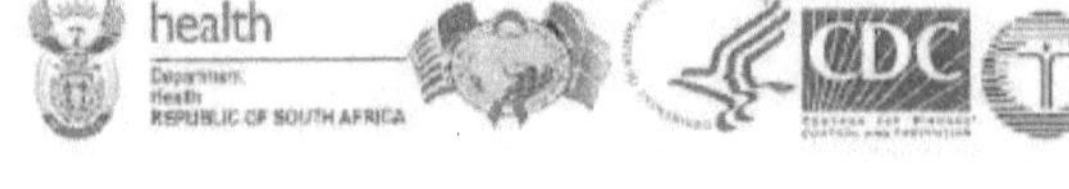
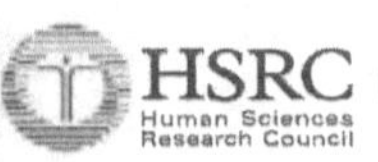
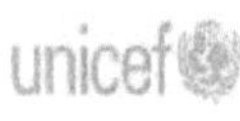
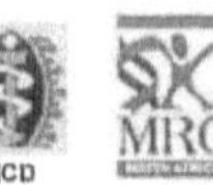

THE FOURTH SOUTH AFRICAN NATIONAL HIV, BEHAVIOUR AND HEALTH SURVEY, 2011/12

A	GEOGRAPHIC AND INTERVIEW PARTICULARS								
Province									
Enumerator area (EA)									
Household questionnaire number									
Person number of respondent									
Clinic number									

B	INTERVIEW DETAILS	Year		Month	Day	Time code	Response code
First visit		1	2				
Second visit		1	2				
Third visit		1	2				
Final response code							

Time code	Response code
1 = Morning till 12:00	1 = Interview completed and sample taken
2 = 12:00-16:00	2 = Interview completed but sample not taken
3 = 16:00-18:00	3 = Appointment made for interview and/or sample
4 = 18:00-20:00	4 = Selected respondent not at home
5 = 20:00 and later	5 = Refusal by head of household
	6 = Refusal by respondent
	7 = Other

INTERVIEW STARTING TIME:

INTERVIEWER: NAME AND NUMBER: ....

C	**REFUSAL PARTICULARS (IF APPLICABLE)**	
At what point did the respondent refuse?		
SPECIFY		

1 = At the gate or door
2 = After explanation of the survey and the process
3 = After the first respondent has been identified (before interview)
4 = During the individual interview
5 = After the individual interview when requested to do the test
6 = Other

Do you wish to tell me why you don't want to take part? You don't have to tell me	
SPECIFY	

<u>Upfront refusals</u>

01 = Too busy to grant interview
02 = Not available now
03 = Too late in the evening
04 = Not willing to participate in any survey/interview
05 = Objected to the topic of the survey (HIV/AIDS)
06 = Objected to being interviewed by the specific interviewer
07 = Afraid
08 = Fear a breach of confidentiality
09 = Government is not doing enough for him/her
10 = Discovered it was for the HSRC
11 = Violence and gangsterism in area
12 = Enumerated in the recent population census
13 = Other

<u>Refusals during individual interview</u>

20 = Objected to providing any/some information on the topic
21 = Objected to providing personal/confidential information
22 = Unable to provide requested information
23 = Refused to continue because he/she got irritated/bored
24 = Refused to continue because he/she got angry
25 = Refused to continue because he/she lost interest or got tired
26 = Refused to continue because he/she was in a hurry
27 = Other

<u>Refusal to provide a blood sample</u>

40 = Apprehensive of blood sample being taken
41 = Against religious beliefs to provide a blood sample
42 = Did not want to know HIV status
43 = Fear a breach of confidentiality
44 = Did not trust the interviewers
45 = Recently had an HIV test
46 = Other

GENERAL INSTRUCTION	CIRCLE THE CODE NEXT TO THE APPROPRIATE ANSWER. IF INDICATED READ THE ANSWER OPTIONS.

SECTION 1	RESPONDENT'S BIOGRAPHICAL DATA

1.1	How old were you at your last birthday? (*Age of the respondent*)		

INSTRUCTION 1.2	DO NOT ASK; RECORD SEX	Male	Female
	Sex of the respondent	1	2

INSTRUCTION 1.3	DO NOT ASK; RECORD RACE
	Race of the respondent

African	White	Coloured	Indian/Asian	Other
1	2	3	4	5

1.4 What is your nationality?

South African citizen	1
Non-citizen (Permanent resident)	2
Non-citizen (Refugee)	3
Other	4

1.5	In the past 12 months have you been away from your usual residence for more than one month?	Yes	No
		1	2

1.6 In the past week, how many nights have you stayed away from home?

0	1	2	3	4	5	6	7

INSTRUCTION	*I am now going to ask you about your marital status*

1.7 What is your current relationship or marital status?

Married (living with husband/wife)	1
Married (not living with husband/wife)	2
Living together, not married (living with boyfriend/girlfriend/partner)	3
Going steady (in a relationship, but not living together)	4
Single (not in a relationship)	5
Divorced / separated	6
Widower / Widow	7
Civil Union	8
Other	9

INSTRUCTION	ONLY ASK THOSE WHO WERE EVER MARRIED

1.8	How old were you when you were married for the first time?		

<table>
<tr><td colspan="2">INSTRUCTION</td><td colspan="2">ORPHANHOOD STATUS</td></tr>
<tr><td>RESPONDENTS
15 TO 18 YEARS
OF AGE</td><td>☐ ↓</td><td>RESPONDENTS
19 YEARS AND OLDER</td><td>☐ → 1.13</td></tr>
</table>

1.9	Is your mother alive?	Yes	No	Don't know
		1	2	3
		GO TO 1.11		*GO TO 1.11*

1.10	How old were you when she passed away? (*Age in years*)		

1.11	Is your father alive?	Yes	No	Don't know
		1	2	3
		GO TO 1.13		*GO TO 1.13*

1.12	How old were you when he passed away? (*Age in years*)		

INSTRUCTION	*"I am now going to ask your employment situation"*

1.13	How would you describe your present employment situation?	
Housewife, homemaker, not looking for work		1
Housewife, homemaker, looking for work		2
Unemployed, looking for work		3
Unemployed, not looking for work		4
Work in informal sector, not looking for permanent work		5
Sick/disabled and unable to work		7
Student/pupil/learner		8
Self-employed - full time (40 hours or more per week)		9
Self-employed - part time (less than 40 hours per week)		10
Employed part time (if none of the above) (less than 40 hours per week)		11
Employed full time (40 hours or more per week)		12
Other		13

1.14	Did you receive any income from any source in the last month?	Yes	No
		1	2
			GO TO 1.17

1.15	What was your <u>main</u> source of income in the last month?	
	Formal salary/earnings on which you pay income tax	1
	Contributions by **adult** family members or relatives	2
	Contributions by **younger** family members or relatives (<18 years)	3
	Government pensions/Grants (e.g. old age pension, disability grant)	4
	Grants/Donations by private welfare organizations	5
	Other sources	6

1.16	What is your gross monthly income?	R					

1.17	Do you have a disability?	Yes	No	Unsure
		1	2	3
			GO TO 1.19	*GO TO 1.19*

INSTRUCTION	DO NOT READ OUT OPTIONS. MULTIPLE RESPONSES POSSIBLE

1.18	What is the disability?	
a	Physical (spinal injury, loss of a limb etc.)	1
b	Sight	2
c	Hearing	3
d	Communication/speech	4
e	Mental or psychiatric illness	5

1.19 INSTRUCTION SCHOOL ATTENDANCE

RESPONDENTS 15 TO 18 YEARS OF AGE	☐ ↓	ALL RESPONDENTS 19 YEARS AND OLDER	☐ → SECTION 2

1.19	Do you currently attend school?	Yes	No
		1	2
		GO TO 1.21	

INSTRUCTION	DO NOT READ OUT OPTIONS. MULTIPLE RESPONSES POSSIBLE

1.20	Why not?	
a	My family does not have enough money	1
b	I don't like school	2
c	I have to look after my younger brothers/sisters	3
d	I have to look after a sick family member	4
e	I failed	5
f	I was expelled	6
g	I became pregnant (if female)	7
h	Completed grade 12	8
i	Other	9

GO TO SECTION 2

INSTRUCTION	READ EACH STATEMENT

1.21	At your school how often do	Always	Often	Some times	Never	Don't know
a	Educators attend classes?	1	2	3	4	5
b	Educators watch children at break time?	1	2	3	4	5
c	Educators watch children coming to school?	1	2	3	4	5
d	Educators watch children leaving school?	1	2	3	4	5
e	Educators monitor the toilets?	1	2	3	4	5
f	Educators make sure no unauthorized person can enter the school?	1	2	3	4	5
g	Boys sexually harass girls by touching, threatening or making rude remarks to them?	1	2	3	4	5
h	Girls sexually harass boys by touching, threatening or making rude remarks to them?	1	2	3	4	5
i	Male educators propose relationships with girl pupils?	1	2	3	4	5
j	Female educators propose relationships with boy pupils?	1	2	3	4	5
k	Teachers propose relationships with pupils of the same sex	1	2	3	4	5

1.22	In the last month have you missed school?	Yes	No
		1	2
			GO TO SECTION 2

1.23	In the **last month**, how many days have you missed school?		

INSTRUCTION	DO NOT READ OUT OPTIONS. MULTIPLE RESPONSES POSSIBLE

1.24	Why have you missed school?	
a	I have been sick	1
b	I don't feel safe going to school	2
c	I don't feel safe at school	3
d	I don't like school	4
e	I have to look after my younger brothers/sisters	5
f	I have to look after a sick family member	6
g	I don't have enough money to go to school everyday	7
h	Exams were done	8
i	Other	9

SECTION 2	MEDIA, COMMUNICATION AND NORMS

INSTRUCTION	*I am now going to ask you a number of questions about different sources of information and what you think of them*

INSTRUCTION 2.1	READ EACH STATEMENT How often do you do the following?

		Never	Once a week	2-6 days a week	Every day of the week
a	Listen to the radio	1	2	3	4
b	Watch television	1	2	3	4
c	Read a magazine	1	2	3	4
d	Read a newspaper	1	2	3	4
e	Use the internet	1	2	3	4
f	Cellphone	1	2	3	4

INSTRUCTION	DO NOT READ OUT OPTIONS. MULTIPLE RESPONSES POSSIBLE

2.2	What has made you take the problem of HIV/AIDS more seriously?	
a	Television programmes	1
b	Radio programmes	2
c	Newspaper articles/ Magazine articles	3
d	Leaflets or booklets or posters	4
e	Billboards	5
f	Signs on taxis/busses/ trains	6
g	Plays or drama	7
h	Knowing or talking to someone with HIV/AIDS	8
i	Caring for a person with HIV/AIDS	9
j	Knowing someone who has died of AIDS	10
k	AIDS statistics	11
l	Talking to a health worker/ nurse / doctor	12
m	Having an HIV test	13
n	Talking to friends or family members	14
o	Other	15
p	Nothing	16

INSTRUCTION	READ EACH STATEMENT

2.3	In the past 12 months from where or from whom have you received HIV/AIDS information that has been useful to you personally?	Received useful information	Did not receive information
a	A child or learner of school-going age	1	2
b	Religious institution/Faith Based Organisation	1	2
c	Workplace	1	2
d	Community meeting	1	2
e	Traditional healer	1	2

2.3	In the past 12 months from where or from whom have you received HIV/AIDS information that has been useful to you personally?	Received useful information	Did not receive information
f	AIDS or welfare organization	1	2
g	Clinic, hospital or doctors office	1	2
h	Telephone helpline	1	2
i	Pharmacy or chemist	1	2
j	Parent / Family member or caregiver	1	2
k	Friend(s)	1	2
INSTRUCTION	Only for children at school		
l	As part of life orientation at school	1	2

2.4	In the past 12 months, which apply to you?	Yes	No
a	Attended a training workshop on HIV/AIDS	1	2
b	Attended a community meeting about HIV/AIDS	1	2
c	Attended an HIV/AIDS play or educational event	1	2
d	Been told by someone you know that they are HIV positive	1	2
e	Attended a funeral of someone who has died of AIDS	1	2
f	Cared for a person who is sick with AIDS	1	2
g	Helped care for a child whose parents have died of AIDS	1	2

2.5	Please indicate whether the following are perceived as socially acceptable practices or not, by: *your peers,* *your family* and *by yourself.*	Peers		Family		Self	
		Socially acceptable	Not Socially acceptable	Socially acceptable	Not Socially acceptable	Socially acceptable	Not Socially acceptable
a	Young women have children before they are married	1	2	1	2	1	2
b	Young men have children before they are married	1	2	1	2	1	2
c	Young women to have older male sexual partners for money, other necessities or luxuries	1	2	1	2	1	2
d	Young men to have older female sexual partners for money, other necessities or luxuries	1	2	1	2	1	2
e	Women have two or more sexual partners at the same time	1	2	1	2	1	2
f	Men have two or more sexual partners at the same time	1	2	1	2	1	2

SECTION 3	KNOWLEDGE AND PERCEPTIONS OF HIV/AIDS

INSTRUCTION 3.1	*I am now going to ask you a number of questions about knowledge and perceptions of HIV and AIDS*	Yes	No	Don't know
a	Can AIDS be cured?	1	2	3
b	Can a person reduce the risk of HIV by having fewer sexual partners?	1	2	3
c	Can a healthy-looking person have HIV?	1	2	3
d	Can HIV be transmitted from a mother to her unborn baby?	1	2	3
e	Can the risk of HIV transmission be reduced by having sex with only one uninfected partner who has no other partners?	1	2	3
f	Can a person get HIV by sharing food with someone who is infected?	1	2	3
g	Can a person reduce the risk of getting HIV by using a condom every time he/she has sex?	1	2	3
h	Can medical male circumcision reduce the risk of HIV infection in males?	1	2	3

INSTRUCTION 3.2	*Now I want to ask you some questions relating to people living with HIV/AIDS*	Yes	No	Not sure
a	If you knew that a shopkeeper or food seller had HIV, would you buy food from them?	1	2	3
b	Would you be willing to care for a family member with AIDS?	1	2	3
c	If a teacher has HIV but is not sick, he or she should be allowed to continue teaching	1	2	3
d	Is it a waste of money to train or give a promotion to someone with HIV/AIDS?	1	2	3
e	Would you want to keep the HIV positive status of a family member a secret?	1	2	3
f	Are you comfortable talking to at least one member of your family about HIV/AIDS?	1	2	3
h	A person would be foolish to marry a person who is living with HIV/AIDS	1	2	3

<table>
<tr><td colspan="2">INSTRUCTION</td><td colspan="4">READ EACH STATEMENT</td></tr>
</table>

3.3	Do you agree or disagree with the following statements:	Agree	Not Sure	Disagree
a	People who have AIDS are dirty	1	2	3
b	People who have AIDS are cursed	1	2	3
c	People who have AIDS should be ashamed	1	2	3
d	It is safe for people who have AIDS to work with children	1	2	3
e	People with AIDS must expect some restrictions on their freedom	1	2	3
f	A person with AIDS must have done something wrong and deserves to be punished	1	2	3

<table>
<tr><td>INSTRUCTION</td><td colspan="4">Now I'm going to ask some questions regarding your general perceptions related to HIV/AIDS policies</td></tr>
</table>

3.4	*Please tell me whether you agree or disagree with the following statements*	Agree	Disagree	Don't know
a	Political leaders are committed to controlling HIV/AIDS in South Africa	1	2	3
b	Political leaders publicly recognise the importance of HIV/AIDS	1	2	3
c	The government allocates sufficient funds to control the spread of HIV infections	1	2	3
d	There are enough community-based organizations helping with HIV/AIDS in my community	1	2	3
e	The government supports people and families living with HIV/AIDS	1	2	3
f	The government supports children affected by HIV/AIDS	1	2	3

<table>
<tr><td>SECTION 4</td><td>MATERNAL MORTALITY</td></tr>
</table>

<table>
<tr><td>INSTRUCTION</td><td>Now I would like to ask you about your brothers and sisters, that is all the children born to your natural mother, including those who are living with you, those living elsewhere and those who have died.</td></tr>
</table>

4.1	How many children did your mother give birth to including you? NUMBER OF BIRTHS TO NATURAL MOTHER		

4.2 INSTRUCTION   NUMBER OF BIRTHS FILTER

TWO OR MORE BIRTHS ☐   **ONLY ONE BIRTH (RESPONDENT ONLY)** ☐ ⟶ 5.1

4.3	How many of these births did your mother have before you were born? NUMBER OF PRECEDING BIRTHS		

| INSTRUCTION | LIST ALL SIBLINGS STARTING FROM THE OLDEST ONE | | | |

		(1)	(2)	(3)	(4)
4.4	Is this sibling a male or a female?	Male..............1 Female............2	Male..............1 Female............2	Male..............1 Female............2	Male.........1 Female.....2
4.5	Is he/she still alive?	Yes..................1 No.....................2 GO TO 4.7 Don't know........3 GO TO [2]	Yes..................1 No.....................2 GO TO 4.7 Don't know........3 GO TO [3]	Yes..................1 No.....................2 GO TO 4.7 Don't know........3 GO TO [4]	Yes..................1 No.....................2 GO TO 4.7 Don't know........3 GO TO [5]
4.6	What is the approximate age of your sibling?	☐☐ GO TO [2]	☐☐ GO TO [3]	☐☐ GO TO [4]	☐☐ GO TO [5]
4.7	In what year did he/she died?	☐☐☐☐	☐☐☐☐	☐☐☐☐	☐☐☐☐
4.8	How many years ago did he/she die?	☐☐	☐☐	☐☐	☐☐
4.9	How old was he/she when he/she died?	☐☐ IF BROTHER DIED OR IF SISTER DIED BEFORE 2000 GO TO [2]	☐☐ IF BROTHER DIED OR IF SISTER DIED BEFORE 2000 GO TO [3]	☐☐ IF BROTHER DIED OR IF SISTER DIED BEFORE 2000 GO TO [4]	☐☐ IF BROTHER DIED OR IF SISTER DIED BEFORE 2000 GO TO 5
4.10	Was she pregnant when she died?	Yes..................1 GO TO 4.13 No....................2	Yes..................1 GO TO 4.13 No....................2	Yes..................1 GO TO 4.13 No....................2	Yes..................1 GO TO 4.13 No....................2
4.11	Did she die during childbirth?	Yes..................1 GO TO 4.13 No....................2	Yes..................1 GO TO 4.13 No....................2	Yes..................1 GO TO 4.13 No....................2	Yes..................1 GO TO 4.13 No....................2
4.12	Did she die within two months after the end of a pregnancy or childbirth?	Yes..................1 No....................2	Yes..................1 No....................2	Yes..................1 No....................2	Yes..................1 No....................2
4.13	Was it due to complications of pregnancy or childbirth?	Yes..................1 No....................2	Yes..................1 No....................2	Yes..................1 No....................2	Yes..................1 No....................2
4.14	How many live born children did she give birth to during her lifetime (before this pregnancy)?	☐☐	☐☐	☐☐	☐☐

INSTRUCTION	LIST ALL SIBLINGS STARTING FROM THE OLDEST ONE			

		(5)	(6)	(7)	(8)
4.4	Is this sibling a male or a female?	Male..............1 Female...........2	Male..............1 Female...........2	Male..............1 Female...........2	Male.........1 Female.... .2
4.5	Is he/she still alive?	Yes................1 No....................2 GO TO 4.7 Don't know........3 GO TO [6]	Yes................1 No....................2 GO TO 4.7 Don't know........3 GO TO [7]	Yes................1 No....................2 GO TO 4.7 Don't know........3 GO TO [8]	Yes................1 No....................2 GO TO 4.7 Don't know........3 GO TO [9]
4.6	What is the approximate age of your sibling?	☐☐ GO TO [6]	☐☐ GO TO [7]	☐☐ GO TO [8]	☐☐ GO TO [9]
4.7	In what year did he/she died?	☐☐☐☐	☐☐☐☐	☐☐☐☐	☐☐☐☐
4.8	How many years ago did he/she die?	☐☐	☐☐	☐☐	☐☐
4.9	How old was he/she when he/she died?	☐☐ IF BROTHER DIED OR IF SISTER DIED BEFORE 2000 GO TO [6]	☐☐ IF BROTHER DIED OR IF SISTER DIED BEFORE 2000 GO TO [7]	☐☐ IF BROTHER DIED OR IF SISTER DIED BEFORE 2000 GO TO [8]	☐☐ IF BROTHER DIED OR IF SISTER DIED BEFORE 2000 GO TO [9]
4.10	Was she pregnant when she died?	Yes................1 GO TO 4.13 No....................2	Yes................1 GO TO 4.13 No....................2	Yes................1 GO TO 4.13 No....................2	Yes................1 GO TO 4.13 No....................2
4.11	Did she die during childbirth?	Yes................1 GO TO 4.13 No....................2	Yes................1 GO TO 4.13 No....................2	Yes................1 GO TO 4.13 No....................2	Yes................1 GO TO 4.13 No....................2
4.12	Did she die within two months after the end of a pregnancy or childbirth?	Yes................1 No....................2	Yes................1 No....................2	Yes................1 No....................2	Yes................1 No....................2
4.13	Was it due to complications of pregnancy or childbirth?	Yes................1 No....................2	Yes................1 No....................2	Yes................1 No....................2	Yes................1 No....................2
4.14	How many live born children did she give birth to during her lifetime (before this pregnancy)?	☐☐	☐☐	☐☐	☐☐

<table>
<tr><td>SECTION 5</td><td>SEXUAL HISTORY</td></tr>
</table>

INSTRUCTION	*I now have to ask you sensitive questions on sex and other sex-related matters. Please remember that your name will not be recorded anywhere in this questionnaire and the information you give will be kept confidential.*

		Yes	No	No response
5.1a	**Have you ever had sexual intercourse?** [*For the purposes of this survey, "sexual intercourse" is defined as penetrative vaginal/anal sex.*]	1	2	3
		Go to 5.3		*Go to 9.1*

INSTRUCTION	SEXUAL EXPERIENCE FILTER

YOUTH 15 TO 24 YEARS WHO NEVER HAD SEX	☐ ↓	MEN AND WOMEN 25 YEARS AND OLDER WHO NEVER HAD SEX	☐ → 5.2

INSTRUCTION	DO NOT READ OUT OPTIONS. MULTIPLE RESPONSES POSSIBLE

5.1b	**Could you please tell me why you have not had sex yet?**	
a	Not ready	1
b	I am too young	2
c	Not interested	3
d	Avoiding pregnancy	4
e	Avoiding STDs, including HIV	5
f	Religious grounds	6
g	Cultural grounds	7
h	Don't have a partner	8
i	No response	9
j	Other	10

INSTRUCTION	*"I am now going to ask you about methods to prevent pregnancy*

5.2	**Have you heard about?**	Yes	No
a	**FEMALE STERILIZATION** Women can have an operation to avoid having any more children.	1	2
b	**MALE STERILIZATION (Vasectomy)** Men can have an operation to avoid having any more children.	1	2
c	**PILL** Women can take a pill every day to avoid becoming pregnant.	1	2
d	**IUD** Women can have a loop or coil placed inside them by a doctor or a nurse.	1	2
e	**INJECTABLES** Women can have an injection by a health provider that stops them from becoming pregnant for two or more months	1	2
f	**RHYTHM METHOD** Every month that a woman is sexually active she can avoid pregnancy by not having sexual intercourse on the days of the month she is most likely to get pregnant.	1	2

g	**WITHDRAWAL** Men can be careful and pull out before climax/ejaculation	1	2
h	**EMERGENCY CONTRACEPTION** As an emergency measure after unprotected sexual intercourse, women can take special pills at any time within five days to prevent pregnancy.	1	2
i	**ANY OTHER METHOD** Have you heard of any other ways or methods that women or men can use to avoid pregnancy?	1	2

ONCE YOU HAVE ASKED THIS QUESTION 5.2 SKIP TO

INSTRUCTION

☐ → **8.13 FOR FEMALES (pg.32)**

☐ → **9.1 FOR MALES (pg 33)**

5.3	How old were you when you had sex for the first time? _______________ yrs old			Cannot remember the age
				1

5.4	In total, with how many different people have you had sexual intercourse in your lifetime?		

INSTRUCTION	**CONDOM USE AT FIRST SEX FILTER**

YOUTH 15 TO 24 YEARS OF AGE ☐ ↓	MEN AND WOMEN 25 YEARS AND OLDER ☐ → 6.1

5.5	Did you use a condom the first time you had sex?	Yes	No	Cannot remember
		1	2	3

SECTION 6	**PARTNER(S) AND PARTNER CHARACTERISTICS**

INSTRUCTION	*I am now going to ask you questions on partner(s) and partner characteristics.*

6.1	Have you had sex during the past 12 months?

	Yes	No	No response
	1	2	3
		Go to 7.1	*Go to 7.1*

6.2	Overall, how many sexual partners did you have during the past 12 months?		

INSTRUCTION	IF '00', CLARIFY THE ANSWER IN Q6.1

6.3	How many male sexual partners did you have during the past 12 months?		

6.4	How many female sexual partners did you have during the past 12 months?		

6.4a INSTRUCTION	Sum answers to 6.3, 6.4 and enter TOTAL		

6.5	Just to make sure that I have this right: you have had in TOTAL _______ sexual partners during the past 12 months. Is that correct?	Yes	No
		1	2
			Probe and correct

6.6	Do you think your most recent sexual partners have had other sexual partners in the past 12 months?	Yes	No	Don't Know
		1	2	3

INSTRUCTION	SEXUAL PARTNERS FILTER

More than one sexual partner ▢	Only one sexual partner ▢ → 6.10

6.7	Did any of these relationships mentioned above overlap with each other?	Yes	No	No response
		1	2	3

6.8	Currently are you in any of these relationships that overlap with each other?	Yes	No	No response
		1	2	3

6.9	Overall, how many sexual partners did you have during the past 3 months?		

INSTRUCTION	IN THE NEXT SECTION, ONLY RECORD UP TO A MAXIMUM OF THREE PERSONS WITH WHOM THE RESPONDENT HAD A SEXUAL RELATIONSHIP WITHIN THE PAST 12 MONTHS If applicable, this will include their spouse / regular partner and any other persons

		Most recent person with whom you had sex	Second most recent person with whom you had sex	Third most recent person with whom you had sex
6.10	Can you describe this partner?	Husband / Wife.........1 Live-in partner .... 2 Girlfriend / Boyfriend not living with you....... 3 Casual partner ....4 Someone whom you paid for sex .... 5 Other 6	Husband / Wife.........1 Live-in partner .... 2 Girlfriend / Boyfriend not living with you....... 3 Casual partner ....4 Someone whom you paid for sex .... 5 Other 6	Husband / Wife.........1 Live-in partner .... 2 Girlfriend / Boyfriend not living with you....... 3 Casual partner ....4 Someone whom you paid for sex .... 5 Other 6

		Most recent person with whom you had sex	Second most recent person with whom you had sex	Third most recent person with whom you had sex
6.11	What is the approximate age of this person?	_______	_______	_______
INSTRUCTION		Insert age of respondent to assist If the partner is younger than five years *GO to 6.12* If the partner is older than five years *GO to 6.13* If the age gap is less than five years *GO to 6.14*		
6.12	What is the MOST important reason for having a sexual partner younger than yourself?	Younger partner is less likely to be infected with STI/HIV....................1 Younger partner will boost me sexually.......2 It is sexually more exciting than having an older or same-age partner.....................3 Fear of getting old; younger partner rejuvenates me...........................4 Having a younger partner will cure me of HIV/AIDS..................5 It is easier to seduce a younger person..........6 Age is not important.................7 Other.......................8	Younger partner is less likely to be infected with STI/HIV....................1 Younger partner will boost me sexually.......2 It is sexually more exciting than having an older or same-age partner.....................3 Fear of getting old; younger partner rejuvenates me...........................4 Having a younger partner will cure me of HIV/AIDS..................5 It is easier to seduce a younger person..........6 Age is not important.................7 Other.......................8	Younger partner is less likely to be infected with STI/HIV....................1 Younger partner will boost me sexually.......2 It is sexually more exciting than having an older or same-age partner.....................3 Fear of getting old; younger partner rejuvenates me...........................4 Having a younger partner will cure me of HIV/AIDS..................5 It is easier to seduce a younger person..........6 Age is not important.................7 Other.......................8
6.13	What is the MOST important reason for having a sexual partner older than yourself?	I feel secure...............1 He/she can support me financially...................2 He/she does not cheat..........................3 He/she is experienced and satisfies my sexual needs.........................4 Age is not important...5 Other...........................6	I feel secure...............1 He/she can support me financially...................2 He/she does not cheat..........................3 He/she is experienced and satisfies my sexual needs.........................4 Age is not important.....5 Other...........................6	I feel secure................1 He/she can support me financially.....................2 He/she does not cheat..........................3 He/she is experienced and satisfies my sexual needs.........................4 Age is not important....5 Other...........................6

		Most recent person with whom you had sex	Second most recent person with whom you had sex	Third most recent person with whom you had sex
6.14	Is this person a male or a female?	Male....................1 Female................2	Male....................1 Female................2	Male....................1 Female................2
6.15	How long ago did you first have sex with this partner?	Days ago [_|_] Months ago [_|_] Years ago [_|_] Can't remember...99	Days ago [_|_] Months ago [_|_] Years ago [_|_] Can't remember...99	Days ago [_|_] Months ago [_|_] Years ago [_|_] Can't remember...99
6.16	When last did you have sex with this partner?	Months ago [_|_] Days ago [_|_] Can't remember...99	Months ago [_|_] Days ago [_|_] Can't remember...99	Months ago [_|_] Days ago [_|_] Can't remember...99
6.17	Are you still sexually active with this partner?	Yes.....................1 No.......................2	Yes.....................1 No.......................2	Yes.....................1 No.......................2
6.18	How often do you use a condom with this particular partner?	Every time............1 Almost every time....2 Sometimes...........3 Never...................4 GO TO 6.22 ←	Every time............1 Almost every time....2 Sometimes...........3 Never...................4 GO TO 6.22 ←	Every time............1 Almost every time....2 Sometimes...........3 Never...................4 GO TO 6.22 ←
6.19	Did you use a condom at last sex?	Yes.....................1 No.......................2 GO TO 6.22 ←	Yes.....................1 No.......................2 GO TO 6.22 ←	Yes.....................1 No.......................2 GO TO 6.22 ←
6.20	Who suggested using a condom?	Yourself................1 Your partner...........2 Mutual agreement...3	Yourself................1 Your partner...........2 Mutual agreement...3	Yourself................1 Your partner...........2 Mutual agreement...3
6.21	If you used a condom, what were your reasons for doing so?	Concern about HIV infection...............1 People are urged to use condoms......2 Want to prevent STI's ....3 Want to prevent pregnancy ....4 Other ....5 ONCE COMPLETED GO TO 6.23	Concern about HIV infection...............1 People are urged to use condoms......2 Want to prevent STI's ....3 Want to prevent pregnancy ....4 Other ....5 ONCE COMPLETED GO TO 6.23	Concern about HIV infection...............1 People are urged to use condoms......2 Want to prevent STI's ....3 Want to prevent pregnancy ....4 Other ....5 ONCE COMPLETED GO TO 6.23

		Most recent person with whom you had sex	Second most recent person with whom you had sex	Third most recent person with whom you had sex
6.22	If you did not use a condom, what were your reasons for not doing so?	Did not have a condom.................1 Partner objected.........2 Used other contraceptive............ 3 Don't like them..........4 Didn't think it was necessary.................5 I am married.............6 I am faithful ....7 I was drunk/high..........8 Other 9	Did not have a condom.................1 Partner objected.........2 Used other contraceptive............ 3 Don't like them..........4 Didn't think it was necessary.................5 I am married.............6 I am faithful ....7 I was drunk/high..........8 Other 9	Did not have a condom.................1 Partner objected.........2 Used other contraceptive............ 3 Don't like them..........4 Didn't think it was necessary.................5 I am married.............6 I am faithful ....7 I was drunk/high..........8 Other 9
6.23	The last time you had sex with this person, did you drink alcohol before sex?	Yes.....................1 No.....................2 Can't remember.....3 (Next partner or proceed to Filter below)	Yes.....................1 No.....................2 Can't remember.....3 (Next partner or proceed to Filter below)	Yes.....................1 No.....................2 Can't remember.....3 (Next partner or proceed to Filter below)

INSTRUCTION	SEXUAL EXPERIENCE FILTER (CHECK Q. 6.19)

SEXUALLY ACTIVE RESPONDENT WHO USED A CONDOM AT LAST SEX WITH ANY PARTNER ☐ ↓

NO CONDOM AT LAST SEX ☐ → AGE OF PARTNER FILTER (Q. 7.1)

INSTRUCTION	DO NOT READ OUT OPTIONS. MULTIPLE RESPONSES POSSIBLE

6.24	Where do you normally obtain condoms?	
a	Government clinic or hospital	1
b	Private clinic or hospital	2
c	Pharmacy / chemist	3
d	Shop / supermarket / café	4
e	Garage / filling station	5
f	Spaza shop	6
g	Shebeen / tavern / hotel	7
h	Other	8

6.25	Is it easy to get a condom if you need one?	Yes	No	No response
		1	2	3

6.26	Did you or your partner pay for the last condom you used or did you get it for free?

Paid for	Free	Not sure/don't know
1	2	3

<table>
<tr><td>SECTION 7</td><td>REPRODUCTION</td></tr>
</table>

<table>
<tr><td colspan="2">INSTRUCTION</td><td colspan="2">NUMBER OF BIRTHS FILTER</td></tr>
<tr><td>WOMEN 15 TO 54 YEAR OF AGE ☐ ↓
Check Q1.1 to confirm age of respondent</td><td></td><td>ALL MEN AGED 15 YEARS AND OLDER AND WOMEN AGED 55 YEARS AND OLDER ☐ →</td><td>8.1
(pg.31)</td></tr>
</table>

INSTRUCTION	*Now I would like to ask you about all the pregnancies that you have had in your lifetime. By this I mean all the babies born to you, whether they were born alive or dead, whether still living or not, whether living with you or elsewhere, and all the pregnancies that you have had that did not result in a live birth. I understand that it is not easy to talk about children who have died, or pregnancies that have terminated before full term, but it is extremely important that you tell us about all of them, so that we can develop programmes that will help the Government of South Africa to improve child health in the future.*

		Yes	No
7.1	Have you ever given birth?	1	2
			GO TO 7.6

		Yes	No
7.2	Do you have any sons or daughters to whom you have given birth who are now living with you?	1	2
			GO TO 7.4

7.3a	How many sons live with you?		
7.3b	And how many daughters live with you?		

		Yes	No
7.4	Do you have any sons or daughters to whom you have given birth who are alive but do not live with you?	1	2
			GO TO 7.6

7.5a	How many sons are alive but do not live with you?		
7.5b	And how many daughters are alive but do not live with you?		

		Yes	No
7.6	Have you ever had a baby who was born alive but later died? (*Any baby who cried or showed signs of life but did not survive?*)	1	2
			GO TO 7.8a

7.7a	How many boys have died?		
7.7b	And how many girls have died?		

7.8a	Women sometimes have pregnancies that do not result in a live born child. That is, a pregnancy can end very early, in a miscarriage or an Abortion or the child can be born dead. Have you had any such Pregnancy that did not result in a live birth?	Yes	No
		1	2
			GO TO 7.9a

7.8b	In all, how many such pregnancies have there been?		

7.9a	Sum answers to 7.3(a,b), 7.5(a,b), 7.7(a,b), 7.8(b) and enter TOTAL		
INSTRUCTION	If NONE, record '00'		

7.9b	Just to make sure that I have this right: you have had in TOTAL ________ pregnancies during your life. Is that correct?	Yes	No
		1	2
		Go to 7.10	Probe and correct

7.10 INSTRUCTION	CHECK 7.9b: ONE OR MORE PREGNANCIES ☐ ↓ NO PREGNANCIES ☐ ⟶ 7.59

7.11	Now I would like to ask about all of your pregnancies (whether born alive, born dead, or lost before full term) starting with the first one you had.
INSTRUCTION	RECORD ALL THE PREGNANCIES. RECORD TWINS AND TRIPLETS ON SEPARATE LINES.

7.12	7.13	7.14	7.15	7.16	7.17	7.18	7.19
Think back to the time of your very first/ next pregnancy.	Was that a single or multiple pregnancy?	Was the child born alive, born dead, or lost before full term?	Did that child cry, move, or breathe when he/she was born?	Is child a boy or a girl?	In what month and year was child born? PROBE: What is his/her birthday?	Is the child still alive?	Is the child living with you?
01	SINGLE ..... 1 MULTIPLE ..2	BORN ALIVE.... 1 (SKIP TO 7.16)◄┘ BORN DEAD.... 2 LOST BEFORE FULL TERM .....3 (SKIP TO 7.22)◄┘	YES ....1 NO .... 2 ↓ 7.22	BOY.....1 GIRL....2	MONTH [ ][ ] YEAR [ ][ ][ ][ ]	YES ...1 NO ....2 ↓ 7.20	YES ......1 (NEXT PREG) NO 2
02	SINGLE ..... 1 MULTIPLE ..2	BORN ALIVE.... 1 (SKIP TO 7.16)◄┘ BORN DEAD.... 2 LOST BEFORE FULL TERM .....3 (SKIP TO 7.22)◄┘	YES ....1 NO .... 2 ↓ 7.22	BOY.....1 GIRL....2	MONTH [ ][ ] YEAR [ ][ ][ ][ ]	YES ...1 NO ....2 ↓ 7.20	YES ......1 (NEXT PREG) NO 2
03	SINGLE ..... 1 MULTIPLE ..2	BORN ALIVE.... 1 (SKIP TO 7.16)◄┘ BORN DEAD.... 2 LOST BEFORE FULL TERM .....3 (SKIP TO 7.22)◄┘	YES ....1 NO .... 2 ↓ 7.22	BOY.....1 GIRL....2	MONTH [ ][ ] YEAR [ ][ ][ ][ ]	YES ...1 NO ....2 ↓ 7.20	YES ......1 (NEXT PREG) NO 2
04	SINGLE ..... 1 MULTIPLE ..2	BORN ALIVE.... 1 (SKIP TO 7.16)◄┘ BORN DEAD.... 2 LOST BEFORE FULL TERM .....3 (SKIP TO 7.22)◄┘	YES ....1 NO .... 2 ↓ 7.22	BOY.....1 GIRL....2	MONTH [ ][ ] YEAR [ ][ ][ ][ ]	YES ...1 NO ....2 ↓ 7.20	YES ......1 (NEXT PREG) NO 2
05	SINGLE ..... 1 MULTIPLE ..2	BORN ALIVE.... 1 (SKIP TO 7.16)◄┘ BORN DEAD.... 2 LOST BEFORE FULL TERM .....3 (SKIP TO 7.22)◄┘	YES ....1 NO .... 2 ↓ 7.22	BOY.....1 GIRL....2	MONTH [ ][ ] YEAR [ ][ ][ ][ ]	YES ...1 NO ....2 ↓ 7.20	YES ......1 (NEXT PREG) NO 2
06	SINGLE ..... 1 MULTIPLE ..2	BORN ALIVE.... 1 (SKIP TO 7.16)◄┘ BORN DEAD.... 2 LOST BEFORE FULL TERM .....3 (SKIP TO 7.22)◄┘	YES ....1 NO .... 2 ↓ 7.22	BOY.....1 GIRL....2	MONTH [ ][ ] YEAR [ ][ ][ ][ ]	YES ...1 NO ....2 ↓ 7.20	YES ......1 (NEXT PREG) NO 2
07	SINGLE ..... 1 MULTIPLE ..2	BORN ALIVE.... 1 (SKIP TO 7.16)◄┘ BORN DEAD.... 2 LOST BEFORE FULL TERM .....3 (SKIP TO 7.22)◄┘	YES ....1 NO .... 2 ↓ 7.22	BOY.....1 GIRL....2	MONTH [ ][ ] YEAR [ ][ ][ ][ ]	YES ...1 NO ....2 ↓ 7.20	YES ......1 (NEXT PREG) NO 2

7.12.	7.20	7.21	7.22	7.23
	IF BORN ALIVE BUT NOW DEAD		**IF BORN DEAD OR LOST BEFORE FULL TERM**	
Think back to the time of your very first/ next pregnancy	How old was the child when he/she died? IF '1 YR', PROBE: How many months old was the child? RECORD DAYS IF LESS THAN 1 MONTH: MONTHS IF LESS THAN TWO YEARS: OR YEARS	Did the child die from diarrhoea?	In what year and month did this pregnancy end?	How many months did the pregnancy last? RECORD IN COMPLETED MONTHS
01	DAYS ......1 ☐☐ MONTH ...2 ☐☐ YEARS ....3 ☐☐	YES... 1 ⌐ NO.....2 DK .....3 (NEXT ◄ PREG)	MONTH ☐☐ YEAR ☐☐☐☐	MONTHS ☐☐
02	DAYS ......1 ☐☐ MONTH ...2 ☐☐ YEARS ....3 ☐☐	YES... 1 ⌐ NO.....2 DK .....3 (NEXT ◄ PREG)	MONTH ☐☐ YEAR ☐☐☐☐	MONTHS ☐☐
03	DAYS ......1 ☐☐ MONTH ...2 ☐☐ YEARS ....3 ☐☐	YES... 1 ⌐ NO.....2 DK .....3 (NEXT ◄ PREG)	MONTH ☐☐ YEAR ☐☐☐☐	MONTHS ☐☐
04	DAYS ......1 ☐☐ MONTH ...2 ☐☐ YEARS ....3 ☐☐	YES... 1 ⌐ NO.....2 DK .....3 (NEXT ◄ PREG)	MONTH ☐☐ YEAR ☐☐☐☐	MONTHS ☐☐
05	DAYS ......1 ☐☐ MONTH ...2 ☐☐ YEARS ....3 ☐☐	YES... 1 ⌐ NO.....2 DK .....3 (NEXT ◄ PREG)	MONTH ☐☐ YEAR ☐☐☐☐	MONTHS ☐☐
06	DAYS ......1 ☐☐ MONTH ...2 ☐☐ YEARS ....3 ☐☐	YES... 1 ⌐ NO.....2 DK .....3 (NEXT ◄ PREG)	MONTH ☐☐ YEAR ☐☐☐☐	MONTHS ☐☐
07	DAYS ......1 ☐☐ MONTH ...2 ☐☐ YEARS ....3 ☐☐	YES... 1 ⌐ NO.....2 DK .....3 (NEXT ◄ PREG)	MONTH ☐☐ YEAR ☐☐☐☐	MONTHS ☐☐

7.12	7.13	7.14	7.15	7.16	7.17	7.18	7.19
Think back to the time of your very first/ next pregnancy.	Was that a single or multiple pregnancy?	Was the child born alive, born dead, or lost before full term?	Did that child cry, move, or breathe when he/she was born?	Is child a boy or a girl?	In what month and year was child born? PROBE: What is his/her birthday?	Is the child still alive?	Is the child living with you?
08	SINGLE ..... 1 MULTIPLE ..2	BORN ALIVE.... 1 (SKIP TO 7.16)◄┘ BORN DEAD.... 2 LOST BEFORE FULL TERM .....3 (SKIP TO 7.22)◄┘	YES ....1 NO .... 2 ↓ 7.22	BOY.....1 GIRL....2	MONTH ☐☐ YEAR ☐☐☐☐	YES ...1 NO ....2 ↓ 7.20	YES ......1 (NEXT PREG) NO 2
09	SINGLE ..... 1 MULTIPLE ..2	BORN ALIVE.... 1 (SKIP TO 7.16)◄┘ BORN DEAD.... 2 LOST BEFORE FULL TERM .....3 (SKIP TO 7.22)◄┘	YES ....1 NO .... 2 ↓ 7.22	BOY.....1 GIRL....2	MONTH ☐☐ YEAR ☐☐☐☐	YES ...1 NO ....2 ↓ 7.20	YES ......1 (NEXT PREG) NO 2
10	SINGLE ..... 1 MULTIPLE ..2	BORN ALIVE.... 1 (SKIP TO 7.16)◄┘ BORN DEAD.... 2 LOST BEFORE FULL TERM .....3 (SKIP TO 7.22)◄┘	YES ....1 NO .... 2 ↓ 7.22	BOY.....1 GIRL....2	MONTH ☐☐ YEAR ☐☐☐☐	YES ...1 NO ....2 ↓ 7.20	YES ......1 (NEXT PREG) NO 2
11	SINGLE ..... 1 MULTIPLE ..2	BORN ALIVE.... 1 (SKIP TO 7.16)◄┘ BORN DEAD.... 2 LOST BEFORE FULL TERM .....3 (SKIP TO 7.22)◄┘	YES ....1 NO .... 2 ↓ 7.22	BOY.....1 GIRL....2	MONTH ☐☐ YEAR ☐☐☐☐	YES ...1 NO ....2 ↓ 7.20	YES ......1 (NEXT PREG) NO 2
12	SINGLE ..... 1 MULTIPLE ..2	BORN ALIVE.... 1 (SKIP TO 7.16)◄┘ BORN DEAD.... 2 LOST BEFORE FULL TERM .....3 (SKIP TO 7.22)◄┘	YES ....1 NO .... 2 ↓ 7.22	BOY.....1 GIRL....2	MONTH ☐☐ YEAR ☐☐☐☐	YES ...1 NO ....2 ↓ 7.20	YES ......1 (NEXT PREG) NO 2
13	SINGLE ..... 1 MULTIPLE ..2	BORN ALIVE.... 1 (SKIP TO 7.16)◄┘ BORN DEAD.... 2 LOST BEFORE FULL TERM .....3 (SKIP TO 7.22)◄┘	YES ....1 NO .... 2 ↓ 7.22	BOY.....1 GIRL....2	MONTH ☐☐ YEAR ☐☐☐☐	YES ...1 NO ....2 ↓ 7.20	YES ......1 (NEXT PREG) NO 2
14	SINGLE ..... 1 MULTIPLE ..2	BORN ALIVE.... 1 (SKIP TO 7.16)◄┘ BORN DEAD.... 2 LOST BEFORE FULL TERM .....3 (SKIP TO 7.22)◄┘	YES ....1 NO .... 2 ↓ 7.22	BOY.....1 GIRL....2	MONTH ☐☐ YEAR ☐☐☐☐	YES ...1 NO ....2 ↓ 7.20	YES ......1 (NEXT PREG) NO 2

7.12.	IF BORN ALIVE BUT NOW DEAD		IF BORN DEAD OR LOST BEFORE FULL TERM	
	7.20	7.21	7.22	7.23
Think back to the time of your very first/ next pregnancy	How old was the child when he/she died? IF '1 YR', PROBE: How many months old was the child? RECORD DAYS IF LESS THAN 1 MONTH: MONTHS IF LESS THAN TWO YEARS: OR YEARS	Did the child die from diarrhoea?	In what year and month did this pregnancy end?	How many months did the pregnancy last? RECORD IN COMPLETED MONTHS
08	DAYS ......1 ☐☐ MONTH ...2 ☐☐ YEARS ....3 ☐☐	YES... 1 NO.....2 DK .....3 (NEXT PREG)	MONTH ☐☐ YEAR ☐☐☐☐	MONTHS ☐☐
09	DAYS ......1 ☐☐ MONTH ...2 ☐☐ YEARS ....3 ☐☐	YES... 1 NO.....2 DK .....3 (NEXT PREG)	MONTH ☐☐ YEAR ☐☐☐☐	MONTHS ☐☐
10	DAYS ......1 ☐☐ MONTH ...2 ☐☐ YEARS ....3 ☐☐	YES... 1 NO.....2 DK .....3 (NEXT PREG)	MONTH ☐☐ YEAR ☐☐☐☐	MONTHS ☐☐
11	DAYS ......1 ☐☐ MONTH ...2 ☐☐ YEARS ....3 ☐☐	YES... 1 NO.....2 DK .....3 (NEXT PREG)	MONTH ☐☐ YEAR ☐☐☐☐	MONTHS ☐☐
12	DAYS ......1 ☐☐ MONTH ...2 ☐☐ YEARS ....3 ☐☐	YES... 1 NO.....2 DK .....3 (NEXT PREG)	MONTH ☐☐ YEAR ☐☐☐☐	MONTHS ☐☐
13	DAYS ......1 ☐☐ MONTH ...2 ☐☐ YEARS ....3 ☐☐	YES... 1 NO.....2 DK .....3 (NEXT PREG)	MONTH ☐☐ YEAR ☐☐☐☐	MONTHS ☐☐
14	DAYS ......1 ☐☐ MONTH ...2 ☐☐ YEARS ....3 ☐☐	YES... 1 NO.....2 DK .....3 (NEXT PREG)	MONTH ☐☐ YEAR ☐☐☐☐	MONTHS ☐☐

7.24	FROM YEAR OF INTERVIEW SUBTRACT YEAR OF LAST PREGNANCY IS THE DIFFERENCE 2 YEARS OR MORE?	Yes	No
		1	2
			Go to 7.26

7.25	Have you had any pregnancies since the last pregnancy mentioned?	Yes	No
		1	2

INSTRUCTION	COMPARE 7.8 WITH THE NUMBER OF PREGNANCIES IN HISTORY ABOVE

NUMBERS ARE THE SAME ☐	NUMBERS ARE DIFFERENT ☐ →	(PROBE AND RECONCILE)

INSTRUCTION 7.26	CHECK 7.17		Number of births
	ENTER THE NUMBER OF PREGNANCIES IN 2006 AND LATER		
	NONE	0	GO TO 7.59

INSTRUCTION	*Now I would like to ask you about your last pregnancy and birth*

7.27	Where was the child born?	Hospital	Clinic	Home or other	Don't Know
		1	2	3	4

7.28	Who attended the birth of the child?	Doctor	Nurse / Midwife (health care worker)	Traditional birth attendant or other	Don't Know
		1	2	3	4

7.29	What was the birth weight of the baby (in KG) (CHECK ROAD TO HEALTH CARD IF AVAILABLE		,
	Source of information (Tick the correct box)	CARD
		RECALL

7.30	Have you ever done any of the following during the pregnancy of this child?	Yes	No	Don't Know
a	Consumed alcohol	1	2	3
b	Smoked cigarettes	1	2	3
c	Used mind altering/recreational drugs	1	2	3

7.31	At the time when you become pregnant, did you want to become pregnant then, did you want to wait until later, or did you not want to have any (more) children at all?	Then	Later	Not at all
		1	2	3
				GO TO 7.33

7.32	How much longer would you have liked to wait?	Months	Years	Don't Know

7.33	Were you using a contraceptive method when you fell pregnant?	Yes	No
		1	2

7.34	Did you see anyone for antenatal care for this pregnancy?	Yes	No
		1	2
			GO TO 7.45

7.35	Whom did you see?	
	Doctor	1
	Nurse/Midwife	2
	Traditional birth attendant	3
	Other	4

7.36	Where did the first antenatal visit take place?	
	Government hospital	1
	Day hospital/Clinic community health center	2
	Mobile Clinic	3
	Private hospital/Clinic	4
	Other private medical	5
	Other	6

7.37	How many weeks pregnant were you when you first received antenatal care for this pregnancy?	Weeks	Don't know

7.38	How many visits did you make to antenatal care clinic during this pregnancy?		

7.39	How many weeks pregnant were you the last time you received antenatal care?	Weeks	Don't know

7.40	During this pregnancy, were any of the following done at least once?	Yes	No	Don't know
a	Were you weighed?	1	2	3
b	Was your height measured?	1	2	3
c	Was your blood pressure measured?	1	2	3
d	Did you give a urine sample?	1	2	3
e	Did you give a blood sample?	1	2	3
f	Were you asked about the use of alcohol?	1	2	3
g	Have you received information on HIV transmission?	1	2	3
h	Were you tested for HIV?	1	2	3
i	Were you prepared for birthing?	1	2	3

	During this pregnancy, were any of the following done at least once?	Yes	No	Don't know
j	Were you tested for sexually transmitted diseases, including syphilis?	1	2	3
k	Were you given advice on nutrition?	1	2	3
l	Were you given an ultrasound?	1	2	3

7.41	Were you told about the signs of pregnancy complications?	Yes	No	Don't Know
		1	2	3

7.42	Were you told about where to go if you had any of these problems?	Yes	No	Don't Know
		1	2	3

7.43	During this pregnancy, were you given an injection in the arm to prevent the baby from getting tetanus, that is, convulsions after birth?	Yes	No	Don't Know
		1	2	3

GO TO 7.45

7.44	During this pregnancy, how many times did you get this injection?	2 or more times	Other
		1	2

7.45	What type of delivery did you have?	Vaginal	Caesarean section
		1	2

GO TO 7.47

INSTRUCTION	DO NOT READ OUT OPTIONS. MULTIPLE RESPONSES POSSIBLE

7.46	Why was a Caesarean section performed?	
a	Previous pregnancy was a C section	1
b	Baby was bridged	2
c	Doctor recommended	3
d	Had complications	4
e	Personal choice	5
f	Don't know	6
g	Other	7

7.47	Did the baby experience any difficulties after birth	Yes	No
		1	2

GO TO 7.49

INSTRUCTION	DO NOT READ OUT OPTIONS. MULTIPLE RESPONSES POSSIBLE

7.48	What were the difficulties?	
a	Breathing problems in the baby	1
b	Bleeding	2
c	Head or brain problems	3
d	Other	4

7.49	Did the baby go home with mother from hospital/clinic after delivery?	Yes	No
		1	2

7.50	Did you experience any difficulties after birth?	Yes	No	Don't know
		1	2	3
				GO TO 7.52

INSTRUCTION	DO NOT READ OUT OPTIONS. MULTIPLE RESPONSES POSSIBLE

7.51	What were the difficulties?	
a	Hypertension	1
b	Haemorrhage or uncontrolled bleeding after birth	2
c	Pregnancy -related sepsis	3
d	Any other pre-existing disease specify	4
e	Other	5

7.52	Did you ever breastfeed baby?	Yes	No
		1	2
			GO TO 7.54

7.53	How long after birth did you first put baby on the breast?	Hours	Days

7.54	Was baby fed breast milk from another women?	Yes	No
		1	2

7.55	After birth did any health care provider check on YOUR health. Was this a ....(READ RESPONSE BELOW)	Yes	No
a	Doctor	1	2
b	Nurse/Mid Wife	1	2
c	Community Health Worker	1	2
d	Traditional birth attendant	1	2

7.56	How long after birth did the first check occur	
a	Same day	1
b	Next day	2
c	Within a week	3
d	Not at all	4
e	Cannot remember	5

7.57	In the two months after birth, did any health care provider check on BABY'S health . Was this a (read response below ....)	Yes	No
a	Doctor	1	2
b	Nurse/Mid Wife	1	2
c	Community Health Worker	1	2
d	Traditional birth attendant	1	2

7.58	How old was baby at this check up?	Days	Weeks	Months

7.59	Are you pregnant now?	Yes	No	Unsure
		1	2	3
				GO TO 7.63

7.60	How many weeks are you pregnant? (WEEKS)		

7.61	When you got pregnant, did you want to get pregnant at that time?	Yes	No
		1	2
		GO TO 7.63	

7.62	Did you want a baby later on or did you want no (more) children?	Later	No more
		1	2

7.63	When last did you have a menstrual period, and can you tell me when it started?
	
	________________
	(DATE , IF GIVEN)
		DAYS AGO 1
		WEEKS AGO 2
		MONTHS AGO 3
		YEARS AGO 4
		NO MENSES
		   DUE TO INJECTION 993
		
		IN MENOPAUSE/
		   HAS HAD HYSTERCTORY... 994
		
		BEFORE LAST BIRTH 995
		
		NEVER MENSTRUATED 996	

SECTION 8	CONTRACEPTION

INSTRUCTION	*"I am now going to ask you about methods to prevent pregnancy*

a). Have you heard about?		b). Have you or your partner ever used (METHOD)		c). Are you or your partner currently using (METHOD)	
		Yes	No	Yes	No	Yes	No

	a). Have you heard about?	Yes	No	Yes	No	Yes	No
8.1	**FEMALE STERILIZATION** Women can have an operation to avoid having any more children.	1	2	1	2		
8.2	**MALE STERILIZATION (Vasectomy)** Men can have an operation to avoid having any more children.	1	2	1	2		
8.3	**PILL** Women can take a pill every day to avoid becoming pregnant.	1	2	1	2	1	2
8.4	**IUD** Women can have a loop or coil placed inside them by a doctor or a nurse.	1	2	1	2	1	2
8.5	**INJECTABLES** Women can have an injection by a health provider that stops them from becoming pregnant for two or more months	1	2	1	2	1	2
8.6	**RHYTHM METHOD** Every month that a woman is sexually active she can avoid pregnancy by not having sexual intercourse on the days of the month she is most likely to get pregnant.	1	2	1	2	1	2
8.7	**WITHDRAWAL** Men can be careful and pull out before climax/ejaculation	1	2	1	2	1	2
8.8	**EMERGENCY CONTRACEPTION** As an emergency measure after unprotected sexual intercourse, women can take special pills at any time within five days to prevent pregnancy.	1	2	1	2	1	2
8.9	**ANY OTHER METHOD** Have you heard of any other ways or methods that women or men can use to avoid pregnancy?	1	2	1	2	1	2

8.10	Where did you obtain (CURRENT METHOD) the last time?	
Government hospital		1
Day hospital/clinic community health centre		2
Mobile clinic		3
Family planning clinic		4
Private hospital/clinic		5
Pharmacy		6
Private doctor		7
Other private medical		8
Other		9

INSTRUCTION	SEX FILTER			
FEMALES	☐ ↓	MALES	☐ →	9.1

8.13	Have you ever had a test for a PAP smear? (By PAP smear test, I mean did a doctor or nurse use a swab or stick to wipe from inside your vagina, take a sample and send it to the laboratory).	Yes	No
		1	2
			GO TO 8.15

8.14	When was the last time you had this test?	
Within the last year		1
2- 3 years		2
4-5 years ago		3
6-10 years ago		4
More than 10 years ago		5
Don't know		6

8.15	Do you have any breast problems?	Yes	No
		1	2
			GO TO 8.17

INSTRUCTION	DO NOT READ OUT OPTIONS. MULTIPLE RESPONSES POSSIBLE

8.16	What kind of breast problems do you have?	
a	Lump	1
b	Pain	2
c	Discharge	3

8.17	Do you regularly examine your breasts for lumps?	Yes	No
		1	2

8.18	Have you ever had a mammogram? (when your breasts are examined using X-rays)	Yes	No
		1	2
			GO TO 10.1

8.19	How long ago was it done?	
Within the last year		1
2- 3 years		2
4-5 years ago		3
6-10 years ago		4
More than 10 years ago		5
Don't know		6

INSTRUCTION	The next section deals with circumcision		
MALES	☐ ↓	FEMALES	☐ ⟶ 10.1

SECTION 9	MALE CIRCUMCISION

INSTRUCTION	*I am now going to ask you questions on male circumcision.*

9.1	Have you been circumcised?	Yes	No
		1	2
			GO TO 9.9

INSTRUCTION	*I am now going to ask you a sensitive question, please remember that your responses are confidential*

9.1a	What type of circumcision?	
Partial		1
Full/complete (foreskin is totally removed)		2
Don't know		3

9.2	How old were you when you were circumcised? (in years)	

9.3	Where were you circumcised?	
At home		1
In hospital/clinic		2
In the mountain/ in the bush/initiation school		3
Other		4
Don't know		5

9.4	What method was used for circumcision?	
Forceps guided method		1
Other device...		2
Don't know		3

9.5	Were you satisfied with the method?	Yes	No	Can't remember
		1	2	3

9.6	Who performed the circumcision?	
Doctor		1
Spiritual or religious leader		2
Traditional circumciser		3
Other		4
Don't know		5

9.7	What was your <u>main</u> reason for being circumcised?	
	Traditional practice such as initiation	1
	Religious reasons	2
	My parents decided for me	3
	Hygiene	4
	Prevent HIV and other STIs	5
	Other	6

9.8	Did you experience complications following circumcision?	Yes	No	Don't know
		1	2	3

INSTRUCTION	ASK MALES WHO ARE NOT CIRCUMCISED	Yes	No
9.9	Would you consider being circumcised?	1	2

SECTION 10	HIV RISK PERCEPTION

INSTRUCTION	*I am now going to ask you questions on HIV risk perceptions.*

INSTRUCTION	READ EACH STATEMENT

10.1	On a scale of 1 to 4 (with 1 being low and 4 being high), how would you rate yourself in terms of risk of becoming infected with HIV?		
	I am definitely going to get infected with HIV	Go to 10.3 ⟵	4
	I am probably going to get infected	Go to 10.3 ⟵	3
	I probably won't get infected		2
	I will definitely not get infected with HIV		1

INSTRUCTION	DO NOT READ OUT OPTIONS. MULTIPLE RESPONSES POSSIBLE

10.2	What are your reasons for believing so?	
a	I have never had sex before	1
b	I abstain from sex	2
c	I am faithful to my partner	3
d	I trust my partner	4
e	I use condoms	5
f	I know my HIV status	6
g	I know the HIV status of my partner	7
h	I do not have sex with sex workers / prostitutes	8
i	My ancestors protect me	9
j	God protects me	10
k	I am not at risk for HIV	11
l	Other	12

INSTRUCTION	ONCE YOU HAVE ASKED THIS QUESTION SKIP TO 11.1

INSTRUCTION	ASK RESPONDENTS WHO INDICATED A VALUE OF 3 OR 4 IN Q10.1

INSTRUCTION	DO NOT READ OUT OPTIONS. MULTIPLE RESPONSES POSSIBLE

10.3 What are your reasons for believing so?

a	I am sexually active	1
b	I have had many sexual partners	2
c	I don't use condoms	3
d	I don't always use condoms	4
e	I don't trust my partner	5
f	I am sick	6
g	My partner is sick	7
h	My partner died of AIDS	8
i	I had an accident / cuts	9
j	Other	10

SECTION 11   HIV TESTING

INSTRUCTION	*I am going to ask you a few questions about HIV testing. Please note that I am not going to ask you about your HIV status*

11.1 Do you know of a place nearby where you can get an HIV test?

	Yes	No
	1	2

11.2 Have you <u>ever</u> had an HIV test?

	Yes	No	No response
	1	2	3
		GO TO 11.13	GO TO 11.13

11.3 How long ago did you have your most recent HIV test?

0 to 3 months	1
4 to 6 months	2
7 to 11 months	3
Less than a year ago	4
Between 1-2 years ago	5
Between 2-3 years ago	6
Three or more years ago	7

INSTRUCTION	*Please note that you should not tell me about the actual result. I am only interested whether you have been told/informed of the result of the test.*

11.4 Have you been told/informed of the result of your most recent test?

	Yes	No
	1	2

11.5 Where did you get your most recent HIV test?

Public hospital	1
Private hospital	2
Public clinic or doctor	3
Private clinic or doctor	4
Mine hospital	5
Traditional healer	6

LoveLife clinic	7
Youth-Centre	8
HIV testing centre	9
Workplace	10
Other	11

11.6	During your most recent HIV test, did you have counselling **before** the HIV test?	Yes	No
		1	2

11.7	During your most recent HIV test, did you have counselling **after** the HIV test?	Yes	No
		1	2

11.8 What was the <u>main</u> reason for going for your last HIV test?

I wanted to know my HIV status	1
My partner asked me to go for testing	2
I wanted to start a new sexual relationship	3
I wanted to get married	4
I applied for an insurance policy	5
I applied for a loan	6
My employer requested it	7
I was feeling sick	8
I was instructed by a health worker (nurse/doctor)	9
I was pregnant	10
Workplace campaign	11
Other	12

11.9	Have you ever been tested for HIV as part of the HIV Counselling andTesting (HCT) campaign launched by the president in 2010?	Yes	No	Don't know
		1	2	3

INSTRUCTION	SEXUAL ACTIVITY FILTER (CHECK Q6.1)
HAD SEXUAL PARTNER(S) IN LAST 12 MONTHS ⬇	NO SEXUAL PARTNERS IN LAST 12 MONTHS ➡ 12.1

11.10	Have you told all your current sex partner or partners about this test result?	Yes	No	No partner
		1	2	3

11.11	In the past six months, how many sex partners have you had whose HIV status you did not know at the time that you had sex?		

11.12	In the past six months, how many sex partners have you had who did not know your HIV status when you had sex with them?		

INSTRUCTION	SEXUAL ACTIVITY FILTER		
NEVER HAD AN HIV TEST	☐ ↓	HAD AN HIV TEST	☐ → 12.1

INSTRUCTION	DO NOT READ OUT OPTIONS. MULTIPLE RESPONSES POSSIBLE	
11.13	**What were your reasons for not going for an HIV test?**	
a	I do not know where to get tested	1
b	I do not think that I have HIV	2
c	I am not at risk for HIV	3
d	I trust my partner	4
e	I was afraid to find out that I might be HIV positive	5
f	I am not ready to have an HIV test	6
g	I was concerned about CONFIDENTIALITY	7
h	I was concerned about STIGMA, DISCRIMINATION or REJECTION	8
i	I was concerned about LOSING MY JOB	9
j	I am concerned about the STANDARD OF SERVICE	10
k	I haven't got around to it	11
l	Other	12

SECTION 12   ALCOHOL USE

INSTRUCTION	*The next section contains questions on the use of alcohol* USE THE EXAMPLE BELOW TO HELP YOU UNDERSTAND WHAT A STANDARD UNIT OR A STANDARD DRINK IS:

One standard drink:

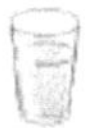 *A single tot of spirits (e.g. 25ml at 43%)*

 *A small glass of liqueur or aperitif (e.g. 25ml at 30%)*

 *1 can of ordinary beer (e.g. 340ml at 5%)*

 *1 glass of wine (e.g. 120ml at 12%)*

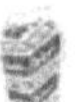 *Carton of ordinary commercial sorghum beer (e.g. 500ml at 3%)*

12.1	Have you <u>ever</u> had a drink containing alcohol?	Yes	No
		1	2
			GO TO 13.1

12.2	How often did you have a drink containing alcohol in the <u>past 12 months</u>?				
	Not in the past 12 months	Once a month or less	2-4 times a month	2-3 times a week	4 or more times a week
	1	2	3	4	5
	GO TO 12.5				

12.3	How many drinks containing alcohol do you have on a typical day when you are drinking?				
	1 or 2	3 or 4	5 or 6	7 to 9	14 or more
	1	2	3	4	5

INSTRUCTION 12.4	READ EACH QUESTION	Never	Less than monthly	Monthly	Weekly	Daily or almost daily
a	How often do you have (*for men*) five or more and (*for women*) four or more drinks on one occasion?	1	2	3	4	5
b	How often during the past 12 months were you not able to stop drinking once you had started?	1	2	3	4	5
c	How often during the past 12 months did you fail to do what was normally expected of you because of drinking?	1	2	3	4	5
d	How often during the past 12 months did you need a first drink in the morning to get yourself going after a heavy drinking session?	1	2	3	4	5
e	How often during the past 12 months did you feel guilt or remorse after drinking?	1	2	3	4	5
f	How often during the past 12 months were you unable to remember what happened the night before because of your drinking?	1	2	3	4	5

12.5	Have you or someone else been injured as a result of your drinking?	
No	**Yes,** but not in the past 12 months	**Yes,** during the past 12 months
1	2	3

12.6	Has a concerned relative, friend, doctor or other health worker ever suggested that you should cut down on your drinking?	
No	**Yes,** but not in the past 12 months	**Yes,** during the past 12 months
1	2	3

SECTION 13	USE OF OTHER SUBSTANCES

INSTRUCTION	*A doctor may prescribe some of the substances listed below (e.g. amphetamines, sedatives, pain medications). For this interview, we will not record medications that are prescribed by your doctor. However, if you have taken such medications for reasons other than prescription, or have taken them more frequently or at higher doses than prescribed, please let me know. While we are also interested in knowing about your use of various recreational drugs, please be assured that information on such use will be treated as strictly confidential."*

13.1	*In the past three months, how often have you used any of the following substances?*	Never	Once or twice	Monthly	Weekly	Almost daily
a	Cannabis (dagga, marijuana, pot, grass, hash, etc.)	1	2	3	4	5
b	Cocaine (coke, rocks, crack, etc.)	1	2	3	4	5
c	Amphetamine-type stimulants (speed, ecstasy, tik, etc.)	1	2	3	4	5
d	Inhalants (nitrates, glue, petrol, paint thinners, etc.)	1	2	3	4	5
e	Sedatives or sleeping pills (Valium, Mandrax, Serepax, Rohypnol, etc.)	1	2	3	4	5
f	Hallucinogens (LSD, acid, mushrooms, PCP, Special K, etc.)	1	2	3	4	5
g	Opiates (heroin, morphine, methadone, codeine, etc.)	1	2	3	4	5
i	Whoonga (mixture of heroin, dagga and ARVs)	1	2	3	·4	5
h	Other	1	2	3	4	5

INSTRUCTION	IF RESPONDENT NEVER USED ANY SUBSTANCES SKIP TO QUESTION 13.3

13.2	During the *past three months*, how often have you failed to perform your responsibilities because of your use of________?	Never	Once or twice	Monthly	Weekly	Almost daily
a	Cannabis (dagga, marijuana, pot, grass, hash, etc.)	1	2	3	4	5
b	Cocaine (coke, rocks, crack, etc.)	1	2	3	4	5
c	Amphetamine-type stimulants (speed, ecstasy, tik, etc.)	1	2	3	4	5
d	Inhalants (nitrates, glue, petrol, paint thinners, etc.)	1	2	3	4	5

13.2	During the *past three months*, how often have you failed to perform your responsibilities because of your use of____?	Never	Once or twice	Monthly	Weekly	Almost daily
e	Sedatives or sleeping pills (Valium, Mandrax, Serepax, Rohypnol, etc.)	1	2	3	4	5
f	Hallucinogens (LSD, acid, mushrooms, PCP, Special K, etc.)	1	2	3	4	5
g	Opiates (heroin, morphine, methadone, codeine, etc.)	1	2	3	4	5
	Whoonga (mixture of heroin, dagga and ARVs)	1	2	3	4	5
h	Other	1	2	3	4	5

13.3	Besides drugs prescribed by a health professional, have you ever used a drug by injection?

No, never	**Yes,** in the past 3 months	**Yes**, but not in the past 3 months
1	2	3
GO TO 14.1		

13.4	Have you ever shared injection needles?

No, never	**Yes,** in the past 3 months	**Yes**, but not in the past 3 months
1	2	3

SECTION 14	HEALTH QUESTIONS

INSTRUCTION	*The next section deals with some questions pertaining to your own health as well services you received in clinics/hospitals or elsewhere. Please remember that your name is not written anywhere and everything you tell me is confidential.*

14.1	Do you do any <u>VIGOROUS INTENSITY</u> sport, fitness or recreational activities in your leisure or spare time, that cause large increases in breathing or heart rate (like running or strenuous sports, weightlifting) for THREE times a week at least 30 minutes at a time?	Yes	No
		1	2

14.2	Do you do any <u>MODERATE-INTENSITY</u> sport, fitness or recreational activities in your leisure or spare time that cause small increases in breathing and heart rate (like brisk walking, cycling or swimming) for THREE times a week at least 30 minutes at a time?	Yes	No
		1	2

14.3	In general, would you say that your health is excellent, good, fair or poor?	
Excellent		1
Good		2
Fair		3
Poor		4

14.4	When was the last time you went to see a health personnel (doctor, nurse, traditional healer, etc.)?	
	Within the past six months	1
	More than six months but not more than a year ago	2
	More than one year ago	3
	Never	4

14.5	Where do you usually obtain health care?	
	Government hospital	1
	Day hospital/clinic community health centre	2
	Mobile clinic	3
	Family planning clinic	4
	Private hospital/clinic	5
	Pharmacy	6
	Private doctor	7
	Other private medical	8
	Other	9

14.6	In the past 12 months, have you been hospitalized for any illness?	Yes	No
		1	2
			GO TO 14.9

14.7	How many times have you been admitted to hospital during the past 12 months?	

14.8	What was the total time you spent in hospital during the past 12 months? (In days)	

14.9	Do you have any chronic medical condition that is affecting what you do or how you feel?	Yes	No
		1	2
			GO TO 14.12

14.10	Please describe this condition you have?
a	
b	
c	

14.11	What are the names of the medicines you are currently taking for the illness or condition you have?
a	
b	
c	

14.12	Have you heard about drug treatments that HIV positive pregnant women can take to reduce the risk of infecting the baby?	Yes	No
		1	2

14.13	Have you heard about drug treatments that can help reduce the risk of HIV infection if a person has been raped?	Yes	No
		1	2

14.14	Are you covered by a Medical Aid or Medical Benefit Scheme?	Yes	No
		1	2
			GO TO 15.1

14.15	Are your visits to clinic, hospital or doctor paid for by medical aid?	Yes	No
		1	2

SECTION 15	ADDITIONAL HEALTH QUESTIONS

INSTRUCTION	*The next set of questions concern how you have been feeling over the past 30 days*

		None of the time	A little of the time	Some of the time	Most of the time	All of the time
15.1	During the last 30 days, about how often did you feel tired out for no good reason?	1	2	3	4	5
15.2	During the last 30 days, about how often did you feel nervous?	1	2	3	4	5
15.3	About how often did you feel so nervous that nothing could calm you down?	1	2	3	4	5
15.4	About how often did you feel hopeless?	1	2	3	4	5
15.5	During the last 30 days, about how often did you feel restless or fidgety?	1	2	3	4	5
15.6	About how often did you feel so restless you could not sit still?	1	2	3	4	5
15.7	About how often did you feel depressed?	1	2	3	4	5
15.8	During the last 30 days, about how often did you feel that everything was an effort?	1	2	3	4	5
15.9	About how often did you feel so sad that nothing could cheer you up?	1	2	3	4	5
15.10	About how often did you feel worthless?	1	2	3	4	5

INSTRUCTION			
RESPONDENTS AGED 15 TO 17 YEARS	⬇	RESPONDENTS 18 YEARS AND OLDER	→ 16.1

15.11 Choose from the list below, the one with whom you spent most time?

Mother	1
Father	2
Grand parent	3
Aunt/Uncle	4
Guardian	5
Siblings	6
Neighbours	7
Person at Aftercare	8

Instruction 15.12	*I'm going to ask you about your connection with the person selected above. "Connection" is measured in terms of the closeness of relationships between you and your parent and or primary caregiver. Does he/she…….*	Not at all	Sometimes	Often
a	Support and encourage you?	1	2	3
b	Gives you attention and listen to you?	1	2	3
c	Show you affection?	1	2	3
d	Praises you	1	2	3
e	Comforts you	1	2	3
f	Respect your sense of freedom	1	2	3
g	Understand you	1	2	3
h	Trust you	1	2	3
i	Give you advice and guidance	1	2	3
j	Provide for your necessities	1	2	3
k	Gives you money	1	2	3
l	Buy you things	1	2	3
m	Have open communication with you	1	2	3
n	Spend time with you	1	2	3
o	Support you in your school work (not applicable if do not attend school)	1	2	3

15.13	Has a parent/guardian ever talked to you about sex?	Yes	No	No response
		1	2	3

15.14	Has a parent/guardian ever talked to you about sexual abuse?	Yes	No	No response
		1	2	3

SECTION 16	CRIME

INSTRUCTION | *Now I am going to ask you questions on crime. Please remember that your name is not written anywhere and everything you tell me is confidential.*

16.1	In the past 12 months, have you been a victim of crime?	Yes	No
		1	2
			Go to 16.6a

INSTRUCTION	DO NOT READ OUT OPTIONS. MULTIPLE RESPONSES POSSIBLE

16.2	What type of crimes have you experienced in the past 12 months?	
a	Robbery	1
b	Victim of burglary	2
c	Car/truck hijacking	3
d	Common assault	4
e	Someone tried to kill me	5
f	Other	6

16.3	In the past 12 months, have you been a victim of a violent crime where a gun or knife was used to threaten or harm you?	Yes	No
		1	2
			GO TO 16.6a

16.4	Was the person who attacked you under the influence of alcohol? Please think about the most recent instance.	Yes	No
		1	2

16.5	Were you under the influence of alcohol at the time? Please think about the most recent instance.	Yes	No
		1	2

INSTRUCTION	*This next section deals with violence experienced in your relationships*

RESPONDENTS WHO ARE IN AN INTIMATE RELATIONSHIP ↓	RESPONDENTS WHO ARE NOT IN ANY INTIMATE RELATIONSHIPS → END`

16.6a	In the past 12 months, a partner has hit me (with a fist or slap or something else that could hurt me)	Yes	No
		1	2
			GO TO 16.6c

16.6b	Do you feel you deserved this?	Yes	No
		1	2

16.6c	In the past 12 months, <u>I have hit</u> a partner (with a fist or slap or something else that could hurt them)	Yes 1	No 2
16.6d	In the past 12 months, a partner has forced me to have sex against my wishes by using violence or threatening violence.	Yes 1	No 2
16.6e	In the past 12 months, I have forced a partner to have sex with me when he/she didn't want it	Yes 1	No 2
16.6f	In the past 12 months, a partner has been violent towards me when he/she was drunk	Yes 1	No 2
16.6g	In the past 12 months, a partner has refused to use a condom during sex, even when I said I wanted to use one	Yes 1	No 2
16.6h	In the past year, have you been to a doctor, hospital or clinic for treatment because you have been injured by a partner?	Yes 1	No 2
16.6i	You currently think of yourself as a victim of physical violence by your partner	Yes 1	No 2

THANK YOU VERY MUCH FOR AGREEING TO PARTICIPATE AND ASSIST US IN THIS IMPORTANT RESEARCH PROJECT.

INTERVIEW ENDING TIME:		:	

Surname and number of editor	

Date questionnaire was checked:	

Surname and number of supervisor	

INSTRUCTION 16.7	WHAT IS THE PERSON NUMBER OF THE PARTNER OF THIS PERSON? (Get the person number from the VP questionnaire)?	

INSTRUCTION 16.8	WHAT IS THE QUESTIONNAIRE NUMBER OF THE PARTNER OF THIS PERSON? (Get the number from the individual questionnaire)?	

Questionnaire number:

Barcode

YOUTH AND ADULT: PERSONS 15 YEARS OLD AND OLDER

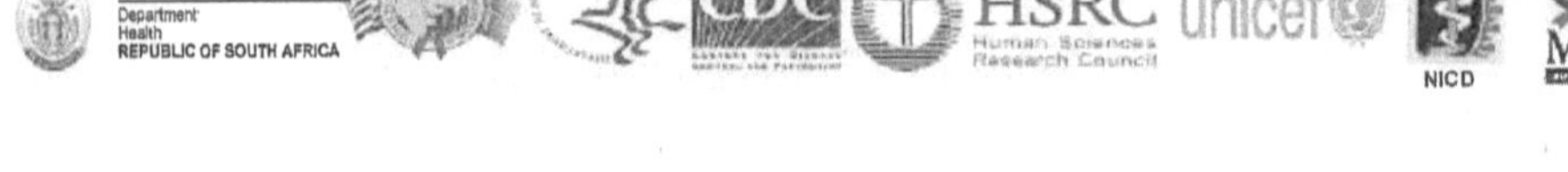

THE FOURTH SOUTH AFRICAN NATIONAL HIV, BEHAVIOUR AND HEALTH SURVEY, 2011/12

Specimen Result Voucher

Dear Survey Participant

If you wish to collect the results of your HIV test please present this voucher to the nurse at the following clinic:

Sex of participant: Male ☐   Female ☐

Age of participant: ☐☐

Date of Collection of <u>Results:</u>   /   /201

If you need assistance call Provincial Coordinator on ...... or National Fieldwork Coordinator on..............

Appendix 4: Ethical approval (2)

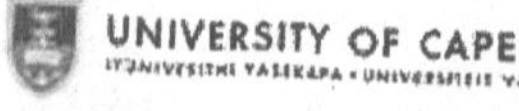

UNIVERSITY OF CAPE TOWN
IYUNIVESITHI YASEKAPA • UNIVERSITEIT VAN KAAPSTAD

FACULTY OF HEALTH SCIENCES
Human Research Ethics Committee

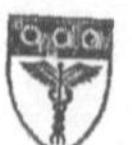

FHS016: Annual Progress Report / Renewal

HREC office use only (FWA00001637; IRB00001938)			
This serves as notification of annual approval, including any documentation described below.			
☑ Approved	Annual progress report	Approved until/next renewal date	30·09· 2020
☐ Not approved	See attached comments		
Signature Chairperson of the HREC		Date Signed	4/11/2019

Comments to PI from the HREC

Principal Investigator to complete the following:

1. Protocol information

Date (when submitting this form)	30 October 2019		
HREC REF Number	462/2018	Current Ethics Approval was granted until	30/09/2019
Protocol title	Knowledge and perceptions about HIV among females aged 15-24 years - associations with HIV testing and sexual behaviour – a sub-study of the 2012 South African National Household survey		
Protocol number (if applicable)			
Are there any sub-studies linked to this study?	☐ Yes ☑ No		
If yes, could you please provide the HREC Ref's for all sub-studies? Note: A separate FHS016 must be submitted for each sub-study.			
Principal Investigator	A/Professor Chistopher Colvin		
Department / Office Internal Mail Address	cj.colvin@uct.ac.za		

(Note: Please complete the Closure form (FHS010) if the study is completed within the approval period)

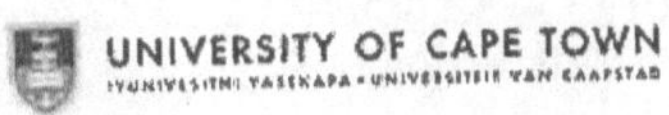

UNIVERSITY OF CAPE TOWN
IYUNIVESITHI YASEKAPA · UNIVERSITEIT VAN KAAPSTAD

FACULTY OF HEALTH SCIENCES
Human Research Ethics Committee

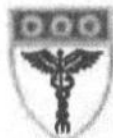

	☐ Yes	☑ No
1.1 Does this protocol receive US Federal funding?	☐ Yes	☑ No
1.2 If the study receives US Federal Funding, does the annual report require full committee approval? **Note:** Any annual approvals for **Full Committee** review MUST be submitted on the monthly HREC submission dates. (Please send electronic copy for full committee review to hrec-enquiries@uct.ac.za)	☐ Yes	☑ No

If yes in 1.2 please complete section 1.3 below for invoicing purposes

1.3 Annual Approval for **full committee** review	- R 3450 (inclusive of vat)	
For invoicing purposes, please provide:		
Sponsor's name		
Contact person		
Address		
Telephone number		
Email Address		

2. List of documentation for approval

3. Protocol status (tick ✓)

☐	Open to enrolment
☐	Closed to enrolment (tick ✓)
☐	Research-related activities are ongoing
☐	Research-related activities are complete, long-term follow-up only
☑	Research-related activities are complete, data analysis only
☐	Main study is complete but sub-study research-related activities are ongoing
☐	Study is closed → Please submit a Study Closure Form (FHS010)

4. Enrolment

(Note: Please complete the Closure form (FHS010) if the study is completed within the approval period)

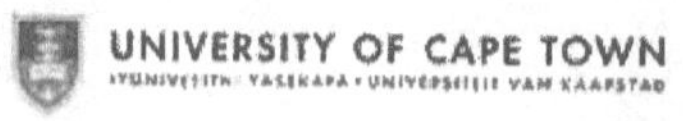
UNIVERSITY OF CAPE TOWN
IYUNIVESITH · YASEKAPA · UNIVERSITEIT VAM KAAPSTAD

FACULTY OF HEALTH SCIENCES
Human Research Ethics Committee

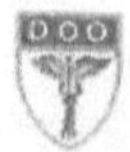

Number of participants enrolled to date	N/A – secondary data analysis only
Number of participants enrolled, since last HREC Progress report (continuing review)	N/A
Additional number of participants still required	N/A

5. Refusals

Total number of refusals (participants invited to join the study, but refused to take part)	N/A

6. Cumulative summary of participants

Total number of participants who provided consent	N/A
Number of participants determined to be ineligible (i.e. after screening)	N/A
Number of participants currently active on the study	N/A
Number of participants completed study (without events leading to withdrawal)	N/A
Number of participants withdrawn at participants' request (i.e. changed their mind)	N/A
Number of participants withdrawn by PI due to toxicity or adverse events	N/A
Number of participants withdrawn by PI for other reasons (e.g. pregnancy, poor compliance)	N/A
Number of participants lost to follow-up. Please comment below on reasons for loss of follow-up.	N/A
Number of participants no longer taking part for reasons not listed above. Please provide reasons below:	N/A

7. Progress of study

Please provide a brief summary of the research to date including the overall progress and the progress since the last annual report as well as any relevant comments/issues you would like to report to the HREC:
The data analysis and report writing phase is currently in progress

(Note: Please complete the Closure form (FHS010) if the study is completed within the approval period)

 UNIVERSITY OF CAPE TOWN
IYUNIVESITHI YASEKAPA · UNIVERSITEIT VAN KAAPSTAD

FACULTY OF HEALTH SCIENCES
Human Research Ethics Committee 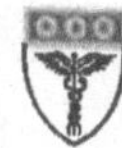

8. Protocol violations and exceptions (tick ✓ all that apply)

☑	No prior violations or exceptions have occurred since the original approval
☐	Prior violations or exceptions have been reported since the last review and have already been acknowledged or approved
☐	Unreported minor violations that have occurred since the last review, as well as significant deviations not yet reported, are attached for review

9. Amendments (tick ✓ all that apply)

☑	No prior amendments have been made since the original approval
☐	Prior amendments have been reported since the last review and have already been approved
☐	New protocol changes/ amendments are requested as part of this continuing review (See note below)

Note: If new protocol changes are being requested in this review, please complete an amendment form (FHS006).
Specific changes in the amended protocol and consent/assent forms must be **bolded**, *italicised* or tracked and all changes must include a rationale.

10. Adverse events

10.1 Please provide below or attach a narrative summary of serious adverse events and/ or unanticipated problems since the last progress report. Please indicate changes made to the protocol and informed consent document(s) as a result (if not already reported to the HREC). Please comment on whether causality to any study procedure or intervention could be established.

10.2 Have participants received appropriate treatment/ follow-up/ referral when indicated (e.g. in the case of abnormal or incidental clinical findings, distress or anxiety)?

☐ Yes	☐ No	☑ Not applicable
If yes, please describe:		

11. Summary of Monitoring and Audit Activities (tick ✓)

11.1 Was this study monitored or audited by an external agency (e.g. SAHPRA, FDA)?

☐ Yes	☐ No	☑ Not applicable

11.2 Did a Data and Safety Monitoring Board publish a report?

☐ Yes	☐ No	☑ Not applicable

11.3 If yes, please identify the agency and attach a summary of the findings.

(Note: Please complete the Closure form (FHS010) if the study is completed within the approval period)

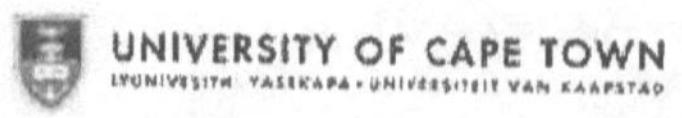

UNIVERSITY OF CAPE TOWN
IYUNIVESITHI YASEKAPA • UNIVERSITEIT VAN KAAPSTAD

FACULTY OF HEALTH SCIENCES
Human Research Ethics Committee

Agency Name		Report attached	☐ Yes	☐ No	☐ Not applicable
		DSMB report attached	☐ Yes	☐ No	☐ Not applicable

11.4 Has there been any agency, institutional or other inquiry into non-compliance in this study, or any finding of non-compliance concerning a member of the research team?	
☐ Yes	☑ No
If yes, please explain:	

12. Level of risk (tick ✓)

12.1 In light of your experience of this research, please indicate whether the level of risk to participants has:	
☐	Increased
☐	Decreased
☑	Shown no change
If there has been a change, please explain:	

12.2 Please provide a narrative summary of recent relevant literature that may have a bearing on the level of risk.

13. Statement of conflict of interest

Has there been any change in the conflict of interest status of this protocol since the original approval? (tick ✓)	
☐ Yes	☑ No
If yes, please explain and if necessary, attach a revised conflict of interest statement (Section #7 in the New Protocol Application Form FHS013).	

14. Signature

My signature certifies that the above is complete and correct.			
Signature of PI	*Christoph J. Cohin*	Date	30.10.2019

(Note: Please complete the Closure form (FHS010) if the study is completed within the approval period)

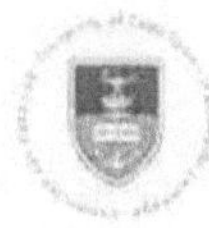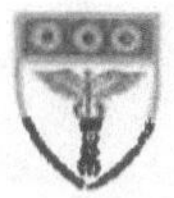

UNIVERSITY OF CAPE TOWN

Faculty of Health Sciences

Human Research Ethics Committee

Room E53-46 Old Main Building
Groote Schuur Hospital
Observatory 7925
Telephone [021] 406 6492
Email: sumayah.ariefdien@uct.ac.za
Website: www.health.uct.ac.za/fhs/research/humanethics/forms

10 September 2018

HREC REF: 462/2018

A/Prof C Colvin
Division of Social and Behavioural Sciences
Public Health & Family Medicine
Falmouth Building-FHS

Dear A/Prof Colvin

PROJECT TITLE: KNOWLEDGE AND PERCEPTIONS ABOUT HIV AMONG ADOLESCENT GIRLS AND YOUNG WOMEN AGED 15-24 YEARS: ASSOCIATIONS WITH HIV TESTING AND SEXUAL BEHAVIOUR - A SUB-STUDY OF THE 2012 SOUTH AFRICAN NATIONAL HIV HOUSEHOLD SURVEY (master's Candidate - Ms Farzanah Frieslaar)

Thank you for your response letter dated 06 September 2018, addressing the issues raised by the Human Research Ethics Committee (HREC).

It is a pleasure to inform you that the HREC has **formally approved** the above-mentioned study.

Approval is granted for one year until the 30 September 2019.

Please submit a progress form, using the standardised Annual Report Form if the study continues beyond the approval period. Please submit a Standard Closure form if the study is completed within the approval period.
(Forms can be found on our website: www.health.uct.ac.za/fhs/research/humanethics/forms)

We acknowledge that the student: Ms Farzanah Frieslaar will also be involved in this study.

Please quote the HREC REF in all your correspondence.

Please note that the ongoing ethical conduct of the study remains the responsibility of the principal investigator.

Please note that for all studies approved by the HREC, the principal investigator **must** obtain appropriate institutional approval, where necessary, before the research may occur.

Yours sincerely

PROFESSOR M BLOCKMAN

Institutional Review Board (IRB) number: IRB00001938
This serves to confirm that the University of Cape Town Human Research Ethics Committee complies to the Ethics Standards for Clinical Research with a new drug in patients, based on the Medical Research Council (MRC-SA), Food and Drug Administration (FDA-USA), International Convention on Harmonisation Good Clinical Practice (ICH GCP), South African Good Clinical Practice Guidelines (DoH 2006), based on the Association of the British Pharmaceutical Industry Guidelines (ABPI), and Declaration of Helsinki (2013) guidelines.
The Human Research Ethics Committee granting this approval is in compliance with the ICH Harmonised Tripartite Guidelines E6: Note for Guidance on Good Clinical Practice (CPMP/ICH/135/95) and FDA Code Federal Regulation Part 50, 56 and 312.

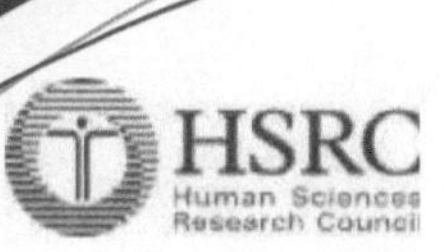

Research Coordination, Ethics and Integrity
(ReCEI)

RESEARCH ETHICS COMMITTEE ADMINISTRATION

Room 1345 - HSRC Building
134 Pretorius Street, Pretoria
Gauteng, South Africa
Tel: 27 12 3022012 - Fax: 27 12 3022005
Email: ksithole@hsrc.ac.za - Website: research.ethics@hsrc.ac.za
REC toll free no 0800 212 123

28 September 2018

To: Ms Farzanah Frieslaar
HIV/AIDS, STIs & TB (HAST)
Human Sciences Research Council
Private Bag X41
Pretoria,
0001
South Africa

Dear Ms Frieslaar

HSRC Research Ethics Committee Protocol No REC 8/19/09/18: Knowledge and perceptions about HIV among adolescent girls and young women aged 15-24 years: Associations with HIV testing and sexual behaviours - A sub-study of the 2012 South African National HIV household survey

The HSRC REC has considered and noted your application dated 14 September 2018.

Approval of the study by the University of Cape Town HREC dated 10 September 2018 HREC REF: 462/2018 is noted.

Exemption from ethics review by the HSRC REC is granted based on recognition of the University of Cape Town HREC Ethics approval already granted and referred to above.

Yours sincerely

Professor D.R Wassenaar
Chair: HSRC Research Ethics Committee

Cc: Prof M Blockman,
Chair: FHS HREC

Appendix 5: Knowledge composite

5.1 Young people: Knowledge about HIV prevention

Percentage of women and men 15–24 years old who correctly identify both ways of preventing the sexual transmission of HIV and reject major misconceptions about HIV transmission

---

What it measures
Progress towards universal knowledge of the essential facts about HIV transmission

---

Rationale
HIV epidemics are perpetuated primarily through the sexual transmission of infection to successive generations of young people. Sound knowledge about HIV and AIDS is necessary (although often insufficient) for adopting behaviour that reduces the risk of HIV transmission.

Numerator
Number of respondents 15-24 years old who correctly answered all five questions

---

Denominator
Number of all respondents 15-24 years old

Calculation
Numerator/denominator

Method of measurement
Population-based surveys (Demographic and Health Survey, AIDS Indicator Survey, Multiple Indicator Cluster Survey or other representative survey)

This indicator is constructed from responses to the following set of prompted questions:
1. Can the risk of HIV transmission be reduced by having sex with only one uninfected partner who has no other partners?

2. Can a person reduce the risk of getting HIV by using a condom every time they have sex?

3. Can a healthy-looking person have HIV?

4. Can a person get HIV from mosquito bites?

5. Can a person get HIV by sharing food with someone who is infected?

Measurement frequency
Preferred: every two years; minimum: every 3-5 years

Disaggregation
- Age (15-19 and 20-24 years)
- Sex (male and female)

Explanation of the numerator
The first three questions should not be altered. Questions 4 and 5 ask about local misconceptions and may be replaced by the most common misconceptions in your country. Examples include: "Can a person get HIV by hugging or shaking hands with a person who is infected?" and "Can a person get HIV through supernatural means?"

Those who have never heard of HIV and AIDS should be excluded from the numerator but included in the denominator. An answer of "don't know" should be recorded as an incorrect answer.

Scores for each of the individual questions (based on the same denominator) are required as well as the score for the composite indicator.

Strengths and weaknesses
The belief that a person who looks healthy cannot be living with HIV is a common misconception that can result in unprotected sexual intercourse with infected partners. Rejecting major misconceptions about the modes of HIV transmission is as important as correct knowledge of the actual modes of transmission. For example, belief that HIV is transmitted through mosquito bites can weaken motivation to adopt safer sexual behaviour, and belief that HIV can be transmitted through sharing food reinforces the stigma faced by people living with HIV.

This indicator is especially useful in countries in which knowledge about HIV and AIDS is poor because it enables easy measurement of incremental